Yin Tui Na

Hands-on therapy for traumatic injury

Dr. Janice Hadlock, DAOM, LAc

Artwork by John Bateson
Cover design by Ben Bateson

Other books by Janice Hadlock, available at JaniceHadlock.com

Hacking Chinese Medicine
Tracking the Dragon: advanced channel theory
Stuck on Pause*
Recovery from Parkinson's*
Medications of Parkinson's: Once Upon a Pill*

* also available for free download at www.pdrecovery.org

Yin Tui Na: Hands-on therapy for traumatic injury
Copyright 2012, Janice Walton-Hadlock
Second edition (revised) 2018

Cover design by Ben Bateson.
Foot bone and arm artwork by John Bateson.

Published by Raja Books, Santa Cruz, California
ISBN 978-0-9979783-1-5

Table of contents

Dedicated to my teachers and to all students of Yin Tui Na and Qi Gong, with special gratitude for the lessons of Sensei Shinzo Fujimaki and Dr. Lee Pu Long.

Chapter one

Yin Tui Na

In Chinese medicine, the term "Tui Na" refers to any hands-on therapeutic technique. These techniques are divided into two types: Yang Tui Na and Yin Tui Na.

Yang Tui Na refers to forceful, overt hand movements such as the abrupt manipulations used in popping a displaced shoulder back into position. Vigorous types of physical therapy such as "bone-cracking" chiropractic and powerful, bruising "deep tissue" therapies such as Rolfing fit under the heading of *Yang* Tui Na.

Yin Tui Na refers to any "light-touch" or subtle therapy that uses the hands. The various gentle, slow, and/or "invisible" techniques, ranging from subtle chiropractic and myofascial release to craniosacral therapy and Forceless Spontaneous Release (FSR) therapy, are all forms of *Yin* Tui Na.

This book teaches Forceless, Spontaneous Release (FSR), one of the most firm, yet least invasive, most motionless therapeutic techniques, as well as providing an introductory version of craniosacral therapy and instructions on a very gentle technique for psoas spasm release.

FSR is a subtle yet powerful way to help a patient address traumatic injuries or pain. This book explains, in great detail, how to use FSR or craniosacral therapy on a person with displaced or injured bones and/or soft tissue.

Sometimes, a person psychologically dissociates from a trauma, which can then cause "failure to heal." FSR brings a person's attention to an injury in a non-threatening manner, and thus is particularly well suited for treating injuries and traumas, recent or long-standing, from which a person has dissociated.

Hey Ma!

Tui Na is pronounced "tway nah," as if to rhyme with "Hey! Ma."

"Tui Na" doesn't translate easily into a specific English term. It is often translated, inaccurately, as massage. A more accurate translation would be "any form of hands-on body work." Literally, *Tui* means push or shove, and *Na* means hold or take. [1, 2]

---

[1] The Pinyin Chinese-English Dictionary. Commercial Press. Hong Kong. 1979. p.698

[2] Although the title of the official Chinese government's English translation of the official Tui Na textbook is *Chinese Massage*, most of the techniques of Tui Na, both Yin and Yang types, bear little or no relation to massage, as we understand massage in the west. See: *Chinese Massage*; Publishing House of Shanghai College of Traditional Chinese Medicine; Shanghai; 1988.

A brief introduction to Forceless, Spontaneous Release

Forceless, Spontaneous Release technique is *extremely* "Yin": firm but passive, often motionless, with no "intention" on the part of the practitioner.

The technique consists of this: the patient's unhealed injury or location of pain is held firmly between the two hands of the therapist, which have been firmly placed on the skin or the clothing in the vicinity of the injured or painful area, until the area responds with some sort of spontaneous movement.

FSR is extremely easy to learn. A person does not need a medical background to learn how to provide firm support to an injured area. A child can quickly learn how to do FSR, and do it very, very well.

The *two hands don't do anything* except hold, firmly, until such time as the patient's *subconscious* mind starts to feel safe enough to pay attention to the area being held, at which point the patient's injured or painful area starts to *move on its own* – often in motions that suggest relaxation of tension or motions suggesting a delayed follow-through and response to the original injury. During these movements, the therapist keeps his firm, supportive hands (usually the palms) pressing on the patient's skin or clothing, while allowing his hands to be carried along by the spontaneous movements being made by the patient.

That's it.

Sounds too simple? It is simple. And yet, much of this book is spent explaining what is meant in the above paragraph by terms like "firmly," "don't do anything," "move on its own," and all the other terms and questions that arise when doing this extremely non-invasive work on a person who has an injury or pain that is not healing quickly *or* who has dissociated from an injury, thus preventing that injury from completely healing.

Another focus in this book is showing the actual hand positions that might be most supportive to the patient while still being comfortable for the therapist.

Still another subject addressed in this book is techniques the *patient* can do to assist and speed up the healing process and terminate the dissociation, if any.

Forceless, Spontaneous Release technique is a type of Yin Tui Na that is particularly suited for the following types of injuries:

Injuries in which some body parts have been displaced, have tightened up and can't relax, or don't seem to be healing on their own.

Injuries from which the patient has dissociated so that there might not be obvious pain, but the area just doesn't "work right."

Injuries the patient doesn't want anyone to touch or even look at.

Recent injuries that are causing pain.

Old injuries that might or might not be causing pain.

Bone medicine

Tui Na, historically, was referred to as "bone medicine." "Bone medicine" in the ancient Chinese tradition refers to both types of Tui Na, Yin (subtle) and Yang (overt). These two types of Tui Na are used, among other purposes, for structural realignment work on bones, tendons, ligaments, and fascia.

Yang Tui Na is used in relatively "strong-arm" work such as the physical repositioning of displaced, *unbroken* bones.

At the other end of the spectrum, Yin Tui Na can be used for painlessly supporting broken bones and/or displaced soft tissue so that the micro muscle relaxes and the displaced bones and /or tissues reposition *themselves* back into exquisitely correct alignment.

The Yin, or "light-touch" techniques in this book were also used historically for *setting* broken bones. Supporting the site of a broken bone with Yin Tui Na can allow any displacements of the broken parts to elegantly, cleanly re-set themselves. This often immediately reduces the pain of the break as well as greatly speeding the knitting of the bone.

These Yin techniques can be helpful and speed healing for almost *any* physical injury or pain, whether new and painful or old and painless. Injuries ranging from concussion or a broken toe to post-surgical pain or pain from a kidney stone that has gotten stuck while passing can usually benefit from treatment with Yin Tui Na, speeding the healing and/or relaxing the area that's in pain.

In my many years as an acupuncturist, I've seen that most patients recover far faster from their injuries or physical pains if some Yin Tui Na precedes the administration of acupuncture. Very often, after the Yin Tui Na work is finished, the pain of the injury is greatly reduced or gone *and* the "channel Qi" (electrical currents in the sub-dermal fascia that give instructions to nearby tissues) has restored itself to its correct pathway – eliminating the need for any acupuncture needles at all.

As an aside, some people assume that the term "Chinese bone medicine" refers to the use of petrified bones in medicinal teas. This is incorrect. For certain medical conditions, including calcium deficiency, fossilized bones (poetically referred to as "dragon bones") are ground up and boiled to make "tea" that provides calcium and other biologically-bound trace minerals for patients deficient in these nutrients. This usage is traditionally taught under the heading of "medicinal herbology and substances." It is *not* referred to as bone medicine.

FSR is a valuable and extremely simple medical tool, one that every acupuncturist – and every person – should have in his repertoire.

Whether you are an acupuncturist, a hands-on therapist, or a support person for someone with an unhealed, maybe even dissociated injury, I hope you will benefit from the instructions in this book. Maybe you will share or write up your own experiences with Yin Tui Na and even post them online. In this way, awareness of this ancient medicine can continue to thrive and prosper.

Chapter two

Dissociation

Our bodies are *designed* to heal.

When a person has an injury or trauma that fails to fully heal, the problem stems from *inhibition* of healing. When an insightful therapist or doctor is working on a patient, he isn't trying to heal the patient, per se. He's trying to figure out why the person's body isn't healing correctly, in the way the body is *designed* to heal from trauma or injury.

Very often, if the body doesn't heal from some painful event, it's because the mind still feels stunned by the trauma or has mentally dissociated from the injury.

The basic definition of psychological dissociation is "compartmentalization *away* from normal consciousness" of some unpleasant event, some body part, or some person or memory. Another way to put this is "mentally blocking out unwanted information."

This might mean that a person doesn't remember an event, or isn't able to feel the actual pain of an event, or might not be able to imagine himself even having the body part that was injured during the event.

The consequences of dissociation from some body part can range from having a body part that's clumsy or "gets banged all the time" or is frequently painful, or hot, cold, stiff, or cramps easily "even though there's nothing wrong." The word "painful," in the above usage, includes *any* pathology, including *painless* situations such as lesions, tumors, numbness, or being subject to fungal growth.

Temporary, short-term dissociation is normal

While a person is caught up in a traumatic event, it is perfectly normal for his brain to temporarily put on hold any non-crucial details, including pain. For example, while running from a lion, a person might not even notice that he has broken his leg. A person in danger might be able to run for miles, appearing perfectly normal, even though a leg bone is broken.

However, once the immediate danger is over, it is also normal and healthy for a person to get himself to a "safe place" or "among friends that will care for me" and then process any trauma that had been put on hold during the actual crisis.

Again, a person in the midst of a crisis might not feel pain or emotion at the time. However, when the crisis or trauma has ended and he's in a "safe place" and/or "among friends," it is normal and healthy for the person to self-assess. He will realize that he's been physically and/or emotionally hurt, *feel* his physical and/or emotional pain, and respond to it, usually with touch or snug wrapping, or maybe even a good cry.

After this acknowledgement of the trauma by himself and/or by others, the injured person's fear can turn off. His innate healing capabilities can kick in.

Temporary, "automatic" dissociation is a healthy response to an injury or traumatic situation at the time of the crisis. Dropping everything in order to nurse the injury back to health right there on the spot might not be wise, as in the above example of running from a lion.

Even very young children can automatically dissociate.

For example, a young child who hurts himself while playing in his room might *not* react right away. Instead, he might silently wander through the house looking for his mother or father. When he finds a parent, he will burst into loud sobs and the injured area will begin to throb with pain.

The child might then be wrongly accused of "putting on a show" to garner sympathy. This would be an incorrect interpretation of events. A child innately *knows* to be guarded and quiet, and to automatically dissociate from pain until he is in a safe place.

For another example, if my dog gets a thorn in her paw while we are out walking, she will not limp or allow me to remove the thorn if another dog is in the area. As soon we are alone or as we near home, she will start to limp again and allow me to remove the thorn.

An animal, after getting to a safe place, will steadily lick or groom the injured area. Fellow animals might join in with the licking. Humans, after getting to a safe place, should likewise put their focus on their injured areas.

The ability to automatically, *temporarily*, dissociate from pain is a normal ability. I suspect most mammals have this ability. (The possum does not. He automatically goes into the immobility of pause mode – the neurological mode of severe shock or coma.) The ability to automatically dissociate from the pain of an injury until one gets to a safe place is a very helpful survival tool.

For that matter, dissociation isn't necessarily a response to a *bad* thing.

A healthy person should be able to temporarily dissociate from his surroundings, as needed, in order to focus. The more focused and calm a person is able to be, the more likely he will be able to dissociate from distractions and focus his attention.

For an example of healthy dissociation, a person who is deep in a book or meditating deeply might not hear the phone ring. A person playing a musical instrument or doing some creative craft might not notice the passage of time. He might miss a meal or two and not notice until he changes his focus. These are just a few examples of *healthy* dissociation.

In my decades of experience working with injuries and movement disorders, I've noticed that the greater degree of self-control, analytical thinking, and word-based engagement with life that a person has, the more likely it is that the person will be able to stay undistracted and even dissociate from sensory distractions while focusing on his preferred subject.

Unfortunately, such a person is also more capable of staying mentally dissociated from negative experiences and body parts, thus potentially making it difficult to fully heal from trauma.

Self-induced dissociation

Some people make a conscious *decision* to dissociate.

For example, a patient of mine told me that fifteen years earlier, when he was in college, he had been angry at his knee because his constant knee pain from an injury was keeping him from playing sports. He commanded himself repeatedly over several days to *not* feel his knee pain.

His command was successful. Fifteen years later, he was in my office with a weak ankle, numb foot, and a knee that kept freezing up on him. In response to my questions, he remembered his college-days instruction to his knees. I did Yin Tui Na on his knees while he worked at consciously rescinding his instructions to his own brain – doing one of the mental Qi Gong exercises in this book.

I refer to this type of dissociation as "self-induced" dissociation.

A person has to work a little harder to destroy a long-implanted self-instruction. It's do-able. Instructions on how to do this are included in chapter six.

Whether a person with a lingering dissociation had a spontaneous, *automatic* response to a trauma but just never got around to addressing it at a safe time *or* is using *self-induced* dissociation as a coping mechanism, like the above patient with the knee pain, the results are the same: the brain will inhibit the person from having access to some or all of the memories or body parts associated with the trauma…until the dissociation is turned off. If some part of the body were physically injured, displaced, or even broken, those dissociated body parts might not be able to fully heal.

Once the brain gets involved in trying to hide things away from normal consciousness, infinite variations are possible. Dissociation is a very personalized brain process – no two people will necessarily dissociate from a negative experience in the same way, if they even dissociate at all.

Sometimes a person is never able to process his dissociated physical and emotional pains on his own. He might never arrive at a metaphorical "safe place" or feel "among trusted friends." In this case, the trauma and injury may stay in place indefinitely. The person has become "stuck."

If a person gets *stuck* in automatic dissociation *or* gives himself a dissociation instruction (self-induced dissociation) and never rescinds the instruction, thereby preventing his own ability to heal, *then* he might, down the road, develop some some physical problem "for no reason," a problem that doesn't heal in spite of treatment or therapy.

The Yin Tui Na technique called Forceless, Spontaneous Release (FSR), can help terminate a dissociation: help a person become unstuck.

As an aside, the word dissociation has *many* meanings. Other meanings include separating oneself from a given individual, community, or religious group. Yet another meaning is the shift in perception that occurs when a person is in a coma or severe traumatic shock (the neurological mode of pause) so that his consciousness perceives itself as being located outside of his body.

For example, many a person has reported to his doctor after his heart surgery that he watched the whole procedure from the ceiling. He can describe in perfect detail what was done and said during the surgery. Unfortunately, from a semantics point of view, doctors refer to this out-of-body behavior as "dissociation," thus giving us two very different medical meanings for the word "dissociation."

In *this* book, the meaning of "dissociation" is the usage I've first described: compartmentalization away from normal consciousness of some event or body part.

Chapter three

About treating Parkinson's disease

Some people use this book in order to apply light-touch therapy across a wide spectrum of health concerns. However, some people seek out this book in order to learn the very specific applications for treating someone with Parkinson's disease. This very short chapter is addressed to the latter group, the people planning to work with someone with Parkinson's. A few paragraphs specifically focused on working with patients with Parkinson's are also included in many chapters.

If you never intend to work with anyone with Parkinson's, you can skip this chapter altogether.

First, Parkinson's disease has a very high rate of misdiagnosis. Brain autopsies show that over thirty percent of people diagnosed with Parkinson's never actually had it. If you have not yet read *Recovery from Parkinson's*, please do read that book, available for free download at www.pdrecovery.org. Please read the chapters on diagnosing Parkinson's, and confirm or contradict the diagnosis, before starting to work on healing yourself or a loved one.

Parkinson's disease is also known as "*idiopathic*" Parkinson's. Idiopathic means "unknown cause." Or you might just call idiopathic Parkinson's the "normal" type of Parkinson's. Parkinson's disease is a *syndrome*, meaning a collection of *symptoms*. The name of the syndrome does *not* suggest a single or specific *cause*.

Some people are diagnosed with syndromes referred to as drug- or toxin-induced parkinson*ism*. In terms of the underlying *cause*, parkinsonism is very different from idiopathic Parkinson's. They are *completely* different syndromes even though they might have some very similar *looking* symptoms. The book *Recovery from Parkinson's* has information to help a person determine which syndrome he is probably dealing with.

Most MDs never bother to distinguish between the underlying causes for Parkinson's disease and parkinsonism. They aren't taught how to distinguish them. Since all symptoms even remotely resembling those of idiopathic Parkinson's disease are automatically – and incorrectly – presumed to be "incurable," there is no reason for an MD to distinguish between the similarly named syndromes.

Second, if you are able to determine that you do in fact have "normal," or "idiopathic" Parkinson's disease, you will next need to determine which of two possible causes is responsible for your own syndrome of idiopathic Parkinson's: dissociation or being stuck in pause mode (the neurological mode of severe shock or coma). Then, you must use the appropriate treatment for that cause.

You will have to figure out on your own what it is you've actually got. Western doctors are *not* trained to do this. Neither are acupuncturists. At least not yet. The book *Recovery from Parkinson's* can help you. It's really not too difficult.

Type 1 Foot injury dissociation: five percent of people with Parkinson's

Yin Tui Na, especially the technique known as Forceless, Spontaneous Release, can be *the* best treatment modality for treating Parkinson's due to dissociation from an injury.

In nearly five percent of the hundreds people I've treated for Parkinson's, using FSR to help the patient mentally re-associate with the injured body part so that his body spontaneously begins the long-suspended work of healing it, this therapy, together with the patient's mental exercises, has been enough to turn off the dissociation and trigger the healing of the injury. This, in turn, turns off the weird sub-dermal electrical schematics that cause the symptoms of Parkinson's disease.

In these cases, the person very often told himself, maybe in childhood, something along the lines of "I don't want to feel my injured foot," "Pretend this foot injury didn't happen," or even, "I don't have a foot." This mental instruction causes self-induced dissociation.

The key point to notice in the above is that the instruction is very specific, and relates only to the injury or the part of the body that was injured.

This type of self-instruction can cause the person's brain to dissociate from the injury, mentally walling off self-awareness of the foot or the injury, as if the injury never happened or the foot doesn't exist. Unfortunately, if the injury "never happened" or the body part "doesn't exist," the body cannot initiate healing of the injury.

Over many decades, the electrical errors in the vicinity of a foot or ankle injury can snowball, eventually leading to errors in the electrical schematics of the whole body. This can culminate in the electrical currents starting to flow in the somewhat bizarre schematics that are *supposed* to flow during coma or severe traumatic shock – schematics that, over the long-term (usually decades), can also cause the symptoms of Parkinson's disease.

In my own experience working with people with Parkinson's, I've had only a very few patients who had *basic* dissociation, as opposed to *self-induced* dissociation. A person who has become stuck in basic dissociation has naturally and normally dissociated during a trauma, but he never got around to turning off the dissociation. He became "stuck" in dissociation.

In these rare cases, the person did *not* give a self-instruction to dissociate. This situation will be discussed more, later.

This book provides instruction for treating both of these types of Parkinson's disease: Parkinson's from either basic (or you might say "automatic") dissociation *or* from self-induced dissociation.

Type 2 Stuck on pause: most people with Parkinson's

Based on the numbers I've seen in my own practice, *most* people with idiopathic Parkinson's, nearly ninety-five percent of my Parkinson's patients, had symptoms that were *not* primarily due to *dissociation* from an unhealed foot or ankle injury.

Most people with Parkinson's, in my experience, maintain the electrical schematics of Parkinson's disease by using the neurological mode of *pause*, not dissociation.

Many people who are stuck on pause are *also* using basic *or* self-induced *dissociation*, but if pause mode is active, that's the more acute problem, the problem that must be addressed first, prior to working on any dissociated injuries.

"Pause" mode is the name I use for the electrical and physiological behaviors that, ordinarily, only kick in during coma or near-death.

Most people with Parkinson's have taught themselves, usually in childhood, to use the neurological mode of pause in order to disconnect themselves from (very often terrifying) physical or emotional pain.

Turning off the long-established, mentally-induced neurological mode of pause is the most effective treatment modality for these people: for *most* people with Parkinson's. Yin Tui Na might *not* help people with this type of Parkinson's and might even worsen their symptoms.

The majority of my patients with Parkinson's gave themselves self-directed instructions, usually in childhood, to "feel no pain," "play dead," or some similar self-numbing, self-protection instruction. Often, the instruction was understood to include emotional pain as well as physical pain. This body-wide type of instruction appears to be met with a very different brain response than the simple dissociation that can occur when a person denies a specific event or body part.

The more-generalized, body-wide instruction to "feel no pain," if given forcefully enough and with grim determination, can allow the person to mentally dissociate from the whole body, very often causing a person to perceive himself as if outside his body, along with instituting other near-death electrical patterns and mental behaviors such as excessive risk assessment and feeling "apart from others." After many decades of using self-induced pause, the sub-dermal electrical schematics of pause can lead to the symptoms of Parkinson's disease.

If a body-wide "feel no pain" instruction was issued and never rescinded, causing the person to become *stuck* on pause, a person with Parkinson's from pause mode who plans to recover will need to *first* turn off this instruction, whether or not he *also* happens to have an unhealed or incompletely healed foot injury.

Pause

I gave this near-death neurological mode the name "pause." This mode is not recognized by western medicine theory. It *is* recognized in ancient Chinese writings, where it is referred to as "Cling to life."[1]

Since ancient times, Asian medicine has recognized that there are four neurological modes: parasympathetic; sympathetic; sleep; and pause. Western medicine only recognizes two: parasympathetic and sympathetic. Western medicine considers the low heart rate, low breathing rate, and immobility of coma to be an extreme variant of "fight or flight" mode.

This makes no sense in terms of spinal nerve and neurotransmitter behaviors, and of course doesn't consider the extremely different sub-dermal electrical schematics of the

---

[1] *A Complete Translation of the Yellow Emperor's Classics of Internal Medicine and the Difficult Classic*;; Henry Lu, PhD; International College of Traditional Chinese Medicine; Vancouver, BC, Canada; 2004; *Su Wen*, chapter 13-9.

"Change of colors [Qi Se] allow for the pulses [changes] of the four phases [modes] that allow a person to be close to the Divine [parasympathetic mode], run from danger [sympathetic mode], [sleep mode], or cling to life [pause]."

modes. Western medicine is only very recently beginning to look at these currents, usually in the research of people who study sub-dermal fascia.

The Chinese medical system's recognition of four neurological modes provides answers to many biological and neurological questions about sleep and pre-death / coma behaviors, and includes the fact that four very different, easy to distinguish sets of subdermal electrical schematics are the drivers for the four modes.[1]

Pause mode is most often used *very* short-term, in cases of coma, *life-threatening* injury, or *life-threatening* shock. As soon as the person has stabilized enough to come back to full alertness, the person might tremor, briefly, and then should automatically, without thinking, execute a series of very quick mental assessments and quick physical movements that turn off pause.

Most of my patients with idiopathic Parkinson's have *lived* in pause mode since childhood.

When a person who has Parkinson's from using pause mode successfully turns off his instruction to use pause mode, then, and only then, if he *does* have foot or other injuries, should he receive FSR or craniosacral therapies to address any injuries that haven't yet healed.

Then again, after turning off pause, treatment of the foot injury(s) might no longer be necessary. Often, as soon as the person turns off the use of pause mode, any decades-old unhealed, dormant injury(s) often become physically obvious: painful, even appearing to be *newly* bruised or swollen. The mind is then able to recognize that these injuries want healing, and they quickly heal on their own, as they should. Often, no additional treatment is necessary. Sometimes, additional injuries do want attention, in which case, FSR is usually the best way to address any remaining injuries.

This book on Yin Tui Na addresses problems arising from dissociation. This book does *not* provide instruction for turning off pause or self-induced pause.

The instructions for turning off a long-held mental command to "feel no pain" or "rise above pain" are provided in *Stuck on Pause*, available for free download at www.pdrecovery.org.

Although nearly everyone with idiopathic Parkinson's disease has one or more unhealed foot injuries, the injury(s) might *not* be causative.

As mentioned earlier, in a person who is merely dissociated from a foot injury, whether basic dissociation or self-induced dissociation, that dissociated foot injury *might* very likely be the *cause* of his Parkinson's symptoms.

---

[1] Most acupuncturists are never taught about the four modes, or even about the constantly fluctuating, minute-by-minute changes in the flow patterns of channel Qi in response to thought, activity, and environment. Although this information has been passed along for over fifteen hundred years in the classic literature, it is not currently taught in schools of Chinese medicine, and has not been taught for over half a century. This is due, in large part, to the modern Chinese government making the concepts of channel Qi and channel theory *illegal*.

This subject is addressed more fully in my book *Hacking Chinese Medicine*, available at www.JaniceHadlock.com.

However, if a person has Parkinson's because he is using pause mode (usually consciously induced so as to block physical and/or emotional pain), *that* usage is what causing his idiopathic Parkinson's.

Most people with Parkinson's are stuck on pause *and* also happen to have one or more unhealed injuries.

A person on pause often does not heal from injuries other than experiencing the crudest forms of healing, such as stopping bleeding and making scars. Truly elegant and complete physical and emotional healing of displaced and damaged tissues is rarely performed *if* the brain is using pause mode, a mode that is supposed to be used when one is teetering on the brink of imminent death.

A person who is stuck on pause may well have an unhealed foot injury: nearly everyone injures or bangs his feet at one time or another. But a person who has commanded himself to "feel no pain" who *then* hurts his foot might never be able to heal from, or even fully feel, his foot injury(s) *because* he's already on pause: unable to fully process or maybe even acknowledge any problem that is not a life-or-death issue.

By the time a person who is using pause mode is diagnosed with Parkinson's disease, he might have a collection of unhealed foot injuries, but they might not be the underlying *cause* of his Parkinson's disease. His use of pause mode is the underlying cause.

Warning

If a person pursuing recovery from Parkinson's is using the mental behaviors of pause mode, he should *first* turn off the mental instruction that is keeping him on pause.

If a person who is stuck on pause receives Yin Tui Na treatment for his foot injury and the foot recovers *before* he has successfully turned off pause, the person may find himself in partial recovery and far *worse* off than before.

He may behave as if his brain is still using pause for *most* of his body but his brain *also* has the *conflicting* information that *some* part(s) of his body, the location(s) of one or more of his recently *healed* injuries, are loved, safe, and healed…even though the rest of him is still trying to obey the mental command to pretend to be at body-wide risk of imminent death.

This mixed mental state can lead to extreme emotional confusion and wariness, and extreme over-reaction in response to unexpected negative stimuli, including one's own negative thoughts. This mixed mental state can manifest in periods of feeling safe, accompanied by effortless, even giddy movement interrupted by periods of *extreme*, hyper-paralyzing symptoms of Parkinson's, much worse than the symptoms prior to healing the injury(s): new symptoms that might last for days in response to a passing negative thought or an event that activates anxiety.

This condition, one in which a person is still using pause mode most of the time despite having healed from one or more long-time physical injuries, I have named "partial recovery."

This condition is "partial" in the sense that one or more injuries have begun to heal, but the mind is *more* confused: at times behaving normally, with no symptoms of Parkinson's, and at other times even more horribly immobilized, and mentally clinging to pause even more desperately than before.

Because of the confusion, most people respond to partial recovery over time by becoming more fearful, and thus more entrenched in pause than before. People in partial recovery often create an "extra personality" or "inner voice," which I have named "the blocker." The "blocker" is a dominating, internal voice that constantly warns a person to *never* turn off the "protection" of pause. The presence of the blocker makes turning off pause extremely difficult. This subject is addressed in great detail in *Stuck on Pause*.

Please note: these weird responses are *not* related to the use of the psychoactive antiparkinson's medications. I will not work with any person who has *ever* taken dopamine-enhancing antiparkinson's medications for a period longer than three weeks. I do not recommend making an attempt at recovery for a person who has used antiparkinson's medications for more than a few weeks.

For more on this subject, please read the medications warnings at www.pdrecovery.org and/or read *Medications of Parkinson's*: *Once Upon a Pill*, available for free download at the same web address.

The two appendices at the back of the book can help you assess whether you are merely dissociated, have self-induced dissociation, are stuck on pause, or are using self-induced pause.

If you, the patient, are merely using psychological dissociation from an injury or body part, the Yin Tui Na techniques in this book will be appropriate.

If you are stuck on pause or using self-induced pause, you will be better served by using the techniques in the book *Stuck on Pause*. You will be better off *not* using the techniques in this book until *after* you have turned off pause.

Then, *after* you have successfully turned off pause, *then* you might safely benefit from having someone use the FSR techniques in this book to address your foot injuries or other unhealed injuries, if any.

I repeat, premature use of FSR or any other type of Yin Tui Na on a person with pause-induced Parkinson's disease might lead to the mental confusion that accompanies partial recovery and even the creation or strengthening of a blocker personality.

I do appreciate that this abrupt introduction of something so weird as an internal voice or "extra personality" may be extremely off-putting to a skeptical reader. However, I have seen this many, many times and have written about it extensively in the book *Stuck on Pause*.

The phrases "extra personality," "someone in my head, " and many others are terms that some of my patients have used in trying to describe the "voice" or "the devil" that's "inside my head." "The voice is telling me not to listen to anyone who will take away my protections" or "telling me it's not *safe* to let go of my protections or even listen to any person who wants to help me change how I think and behave."

This "voice" usually appears in response to doing therapeutical work such as FSR on injuries *prior* to turning off pause.

It can be much, much harder to turn off pause if a blocker personality has been activated.

Please, do not use Yin Tui Na therapy on a person with Parkinson's disease who is using pause mode.

Again, the appendices can help you assess whether a person is merely dissociated, have self-induced dissociation, are stuck on pause, or are using self-induced pause.

Also, redundantly, *before* working with a patient with Parkinson's, please read the warning about attempting to recover after having used dopamine-enhancing medications for more than three weeks. This medications warning is posted on the website of the Parkinson's Recovery Project: www.pdrecovery.org.

Chapter four

Yin Tui Na: overview of techniques

1) The first therapeutic techniques discussed in this book are the mental therapies that the patient can perform by himself. This can be done *while* receiving physical Yin Tui Na treatments *or* during one's spare time.

Techniques of mental medical Qi Gong can help the patient in re-associating with a dissociated body part, greatly accelerating healing. "Qi Gong" literally means "energy control." Mental medical Qi Gong is the general name for healing protocols that encourage or destroy certain thought patterns. For example, the widely practiced, extremely helpful modern technique of "cognitive behavioral therapy" can be considered, in Chinese medicine, a type of mental medical Qi Gong.

Qi Gong techniques that can help eliminate a dissociation pattern in the brain are taught in chapters five and six.

2) The second technique discussed in this book, Forceless, Spontaneous Release, or FSR, instructs in a certain *tempo* of treatment (slow), amount of *pressure* applied with one's hands (firm), and the *lack* of intention that the practitioner brings to the treatment. The physical and emotional support provided by this technique can bring a patient's attention to an injured area so that healing can begin.

The comforting effect of "firm but passive" is similar to the deeply soothing comfort given to an infant by firm, tight swaddling.

This technique does *not* apply particular vectors, force in specific *directions* of movement, to the patient. However, corrective movement in twisted or displaced tissues often occurs, spontaneously, as the patient responds to the firm support.

This technique can also be used diagnostically, to detect injuries and pathological holding patterns in the body.

FSR can be performed anywhere on the body that has unhealed injuries. In people with Parkinson's from dissociation, the legs, feet, and ankles are areas that nearly always call out for treatment, but there may be other injured areas, as well.

3) The third technique discussed uses extremely gentle nudges to suggest directional movements in muscles that have become stuck in a particular holding pattern.

This technique of gentle nudges can be used in almost any body part that has become locked up. This book has examples of this technique, including examples for rotational joints of the hips and shoulders. This particular technique of "gentle nudging" does not have a name. It uses the tempo and support principles of FSR, but has intentional movement.

4) The fourth technique, craniosacral therapy, is a method for restoring and/or improving the flow of cerebrospinal fluid via correcting displaced cranial and spinal bones or turning off micro-muscle holding patterns in the joints of these bones. To assist in healthy movement of cerebrospinal fluid, gentle, directional pressures are applied at the various cranial and spinal joint articulations. (An articulation is a meeting point between bones that move.) The vectors for the induced movements at these articulations are highly specific, and are aimed at maximizing the openness of these joints.

This book describes the hand positions and some of the possible vector directions most commonly used in craniosacral therapy.

When treating craniosacral injuries from which a person has become dissociated, you should *not* use the tempo, amount of pressure, or the degree of intention that is typically taught in craniosacral protocols. Instead, in these patients, the very specific hand placements of craniosacral therapy are best combined with the FSR tempo, degree of hand pressure, and a *lack* of direction and intention.

Instead of the usual craniosacral therapy directional forces, a very firm but much more passive approach is used while gaining the trust of a brain that's been automatically dissociated from a trauma *or* that has been consciously *instructed* to dissociate.

Many health practitioners consider the directional nudging used in most styles of craniosacral therapy to be extremely minimal and non-invasive. However, even this very small amount of forced movement is often perceived as manipulative and threatening by many people who are dissociated, on pause, or who have Parkinson's. Using FSR guidelines while using the various craniosacral hand positions is *much* less invasive than traditional craniosacral work and much more likely to lead to re-association with the restricted area (if dissociated), and/or the release of tension in a post-injury holding pattern.

5) The fifth technique in this book instructs in an extremely gentle, or "Yin" technique for releasing psoas muscle spasms – a spasm that is not uncommon in people with conditions ranging from ear ringing or back pain to Parkinson's disease.

Many techniques have been developed for releasing psoas muscle spasms. Some of them are quite forceful. The very Yin method of psoas release taught herein, which people can do on themselves, is very soothing. Unlike the painful, forceful, and even brutal methods for forcing the release of a psoas spasm, this gentle approach is simple and painless.

6) In the appendix are two chapters lifted from the book *Stuck on Pause* to help you determine whether you are using dissociation or pause. Before starting to use the Yin Tui Na techniques in this book, please read about and perform the diagnostic tests in the appendix.

If you determine that you *are* dissociated and, for people with Parkinson's, that you are *not* stuck on pause, feel free to jump into the next chapter to start work on turning off the dissociation.

Chapter five

Turning off dissociation: medical Qi Gong

Yin Tui Na therapy can promote healing *and* can help turn off dissociation. Turning off dissociation can be *greatly* accelerated if the patient does certain mental techniques during his Yin Tui Na treatment *or* at any other time. In the field of Chinese medicine, this type of mind-work is referred to as mental medical Qi Gong.

This chapter will teach the mental exercises a person can do to help turn off dissociation. The chapter *after* this one teaches the exercises for turning off *self-induced* dissociation.

By the way, not everyone with an injury has necessarily dissociated from it or is stuck on pause. Please visit the appendices to determine if you have dissociated from an injury.

Think of dissociation as an instruction in your mind that forbids you having access to some particular bit of brain information, information that has been stored in your brain's "Events Memory" area and/or your "Somatic Awareness of Body Parts" area. The information is there, but it's been sealed off.

The goal in turning *off* dissociation is to destroy or re-route the brain cell (neuron) "walls" or "bypasses" that your brain constructed to block off these areas. The information is still in there. It's just walled off. If you like, you can imagine that a brain cell has been instructed to serve as a moat around the negative memory, making it inaccessible. The techniques in this chapter will explain how to destroy that "wall" or "moat" or whatever visual image or story line you've created in order to block access. You have the right to regain access to your own mental history.

The light and energy technique

Lie down and relax.

If you already jumped ahead to the appendix to determine whether you are using dissociation or pause, you will already know that, when visualizing injured areas in your own body, the areas that are imagined to be dark and *motionless* are dissociated and those that appear dark and agitated are stuck on pause.

If you haven't already read the appendix, take a moment right now to read the material on pages 169 to 171, the basic introduction to making a diagnosis of dissociation. That material will explain what's meant by "looking around inside" and "easier to imagine as light or dark."

After you've read this material, you will start the light and energy technique by doing the same type of diagnostic exercises that is explained in Appendix I: Diagnosing dissociation.

You will mentally explore inside your body, noticing if various areas are easier to imagine as dark or as filled with light.

As with the diagnostic exercises in that appendix, start with light in your nose, and then move on to other areas until you are ready to home in on the problem area. The problem area, as you have probably already noticed while making a diagnosis of dissociation, is dark and heavy, or dark and *immobilized*: not moving. It might also be so dark and immobile that it's impossible to imagine.

Gaze at this most-dark area inside your body: at the area that is dark, cloudy, gray or even "non-existent."

Focus on the very *center* of this area: the area that is darkest, least visible or that you least *want* to look at or are least *able* to look at.

When you've found the "darkest" spot, that's the area you want to work on. Imagine a small dot of bright, white, laser light right in the very center of the area that your brain doesn't want you to access. Hold this light for a count of ten. Then relax and let the light turn off.

The light should be small: smaller than a lentil, bigger than the head of a pin, if possible. If all you can get is a fleeting spark, fine. Start with that.

If possible, in addition to the bright light, you may also send a *tiny* bit of muscle tone to the area. Not enough muscle tone to actually tighten or clench a muscle, but just enough to make your brain think a bit about increasing energy to the area. This can make the re-connection go faster.

However, if you have some emotional reluctance to imagining a few milliwatts of energy going to this area, then don't do it. In general, if there is pain in the area, only send a small amount of energy. The greater the amount of physical pain, the less physical energy you want to send to the area. If the area is in a *lot* of pain, as it might be if you have just broken a bone, don't send muscle-tightening energy. Just send light.

Only the very center

Do *not* send light or muscle tension to the *entire* area or the periphery. Just send it to the very *center* of the dissociated area. Isolating the *core* of the problem area will force your brain to grudgingly allow access to the exact spot it is trying to avoid.

Next, you will repeat, nine more times, the technique of "bright light and maybe muscle tone to a count of ten."

You already did one set of ten. When you complete nine more sets, you'll have done ten sets. Ten sets, each one to a count of ten. A total of one hundred counts.

After your first attempt to hold light for a count of ten, but *before* jumping in and doing the remaining nine sets, first take a moment to talk to your brain.

You might want to silently say thank you to your brain for having protected you from awareness of pain, as requested at some time in the past.

Then tell your mind, "Now it's time to end that. I'm safe now. I'm going to re-connect with the areas that are dissociated."

Be firm but loving and understanding. Your brain might not trust that you are sincere or that you are safe, at first, or it might be reluctant to abandon old habits. This isn't a "bad" thing. This is just how brains and habits work.

After having established that you are, in fact, going to re-connect with the dissociated area, repeat the "white light, hold for a count of ten, maybe use slight muscle tone in the exact center of the area – and *none* in the perpiphery," nine more times.

That's it. That's the technique.

When you are finished with ten sets, mentally look around inside and see if the dark area is changing: getting darker, lighter, becoming even more motionless, changing to agitated, or feeling more lively or "connected" to the rest of your body.

If it is still dark and immobile, do this technique again, maybe two or three more times.

If it is still dark but now, in your imagination or visualization, the area appears to be microscopically *trembling* or visibly *agitated* in *any* way (as opposed to locked down and immobilized, or happily connected), you may well have exposed (opened the curtains of awareness in) an area that is in shock. Very likely, in the past, you dissociated from the signals telling you that you were in shock but those agitated on-pause signals are still there, running in the background. Now that the dissociation is gone, the agitated pause-mode behaviors (from shock) are exposed.

If this is the case, you will want do the steps for turning off pause. These are explained in the book *Stuck on Pause.*[1]

It is not uncommon for an area that presents as dark and immobile (dissociated) to be masking an area that is dark agitated (on pause). It is also not uncommon to see the opposite: an agitated area that, when the agitation is turned off, becomes dark and immobile.

Treat whatever situation is presenting at the moment.

If the presentation changes, then treat the new presentation. These multiple layers of self-protection barriers can develop when a person either dissociates from an area that's already stuck in shock (stuck on pause) or the reverse: he has dissociated from some area that subsequently is violently traumatized and gets stuck on pause – but he can't come out of shock because the area is inaccessible to his mind from having previously dissociated.

A person who uses his brain instead of his somatic awareness to deal with injury and trauma can build multiple layers of denial. Again, treat whatever situation, either dissociation or pause, that is presenting at the moment.

Self-induced dissociation

If the darkness is lighter for a short duration after doing the light and energy technique *but* gets dark again or the dark area starts moving around and/or acting evasive, you most likely will need to follow the instructions in the next chapter for turning off *self-induced* dissociation.

If, after ten sets (one "session"), or maybe a few more sessions, the dark area gets lighter and *stays* lighter, and is still lighter the next day, congratulate yourself and maybe blow the previously dark area a mental kiss.

---

[1] Available for free download at www.pdrecovery.org, in the Publications section. It is also available at www.JaniceHadlock.com.

You only need to do a re-association technique until the area is easier to imagine being light and full of life instead of dark and immobile. Once the area is *consistently* light and feels as if it's a part of you, you don't need to do this anymore.

Watch out for the detour

Very often, the brain will not want to comply with the light and energy technique. After all, you once told yourself that you aren't safe yet or you made some other self-protection comment that caused your brain to stay dissociated from the trauma.

While you are trying to do ten sets of this exercise, your thoughts might suddenly wander. You may find yourself silently saying something like, "What's for dinner tonight?" or "What should I wear tomorrow?"

This self-distraction ploy is extremely common. I would guess that around ninety percent of my patients have experienced it.

If you notice your brain trying to distract you from the job at hand, just lovingly refocus back into what you are doing: a small spot of bright light, hold it for a count of ten. Repeat.

After all, who's in charge here? Your conscious mind or your stodgy brain habits? With increased determination, love, and compassion for yourself, finish your ten sets of counting to ten.

The brain's attempt at a mental detour usually occurs around the 5th, 6th, or 7th set, right around the time that you are about to successfully modify your brain's neural behavior. However, it can occur at any point in the process. Don't be angry with your brain. It's trying to comply with what it thinks you want, based on your days, weeks, or years of the dissociation habit.

I can't do this

If you can't imagine even this small amount of light, just do the best you can.

If you can only imagine colored light, fine. Keep at it, and you will soon enough be able to imagine white light.

If the light flickers or comes and goes, fine. Stick with it.

Do not worry about making it perfect in the beginning. You are changing a long-term habit. It may take several repeats of the technique or even several attempts spread out over a few hours or several days. *Don't* be obsessively worried about it. If what you have is simple, automatic dissociation that was never turned off, the brain will change fairly soon in response to this technique.

Do this technique with loving understanding, maybe even with a sense of humor. Don't do it with grim determination.

If the problem doesn't resolve or keeps returning

The very nature of the brain is to be obedient to your instructions. If you stick to your new intention, your brain will rally round and make the re-connection changes you desire *if* it is allowed to, according to the laws of biology and psychology.

If your brain *doesn't* make lasting change in response to the light and energy technique, you are probably using *self-induced* dissociation, which requires a different treatment technique – one described in the next chapter.

If the dark area(s) change locations, or are restored to "light" and "alive," *but* resume darkness and immobility sometime later, or have some new weird and unhealthy presentation in a few minutes or in an hour or so, or in a few days, you may have self-induced dissociation. You may have *consciously* commanded yourself to not ever feel or be aware of that body part or event.

You will need to destroy the brain instruction instead of just re-connecting with the inaccessible area.

Again, redundantly, if this is the case, you will want to use the technique discussed in the next chapter.

My introduction to focusing on pain

Back in my undergraduate college days, I banged my head on an open kitchen cabinet door and yelped. I caught my breath and told my concerned housemate, "Don't worry, I'll just distract myself. If I think of something else, I won't feel the pain."

She drawled, "You know, In *China*, they *focus* on the area when it gets hurt. They don't try to *avoid* it."

This was before president Nixon's famous visit to China in 1972. For decades prior to this visit, China had been a locked box to Americans. For Americans, anything having to do with China was cloaked in mystery. One could say *anything* about China and have some number of believers.

I snapped back, "Well that's just stupid! Why would anyone want to make the pain *worse*?"

I didn't know then that pain from injury is usually just a message to the brain saying, "Hey, we might have a problem here. Will you take a look at it?"

If the mind responds by calmly *observing* the painful area, the pain level quickly drops. And if the observation is followed up by sending energy and love into the injured area, the area can heal *much* faster than if it is ignored or denied.

Filling an injured area with light and/or power is an ancient, eastern way of quickly activating healing and reducing pain in an injury. The light and energy technique is an ideal way for *immediately* dealing with injuries. It is the *opposite* of dissociating from them and waiting for a more convenient time to do your healing, if ever. [1]

Yet another method: installing a beloved

Another ancient and elegant technique for dealing with an injury is imagining someone – any inspirational figure who is trusted and loved – being miniaturized and allowed into the injury site. Once there, he/she/it stays there, filling the area with warmth and light. You can talk to the figure or just gaze at it. The more you engage with the beloved figure that is sitting there sweetly in the middle of the injury area, the faster the injury will heal.

---

[1] I learned this yogic "light and energy, count to ten" technique, which is also a form of medical Qi Gong if you prefer to think in terms of Chinese rather than yogic protocols, in the late 1980s, from materials written by Paramahansa Yogananda (1893-1952). I do not recall the title of the book or article that shared this information.

The beloved does not serve as protection *against* the problem area. Just the opposite. He/she serves as your guide *into* the problem area. You give permission for your loved one to fill the area with warmth, light, and love and you *pay attention* to him/her.

Because you love being with and communicating with your friend, you are happy to watch/feel energy, light, and love flowing into the area that you've injured or from which you might have dissociated. Your loved one is there to hold your hand as you focus on the area.

You can do this until the darkness lightens up or the sharp pain, if any, starts to climb down. Or you can keep your friend there until the area is completely healed.

For that matter, some people keep a mental image of a loved one in the area of their physical heart at all times.

Busy miners with helmet lights

If you need to have helpers that are more dynamic than just a statuesque figure ensconced in your injury, you can try this one:

This method was used by a highly respected Buddhist teacher whose name, sadly, I do not recall. I learned of this method decades ago, from one of his students.

The teacher's hand had been badly smashed in an accident. The doctors wanted to amputate before gangrene set in. He asked for three days to work on it before they cut it off.

He spent the next three days in solitude, imagining work crews of tiny miners marching into and out of his hand. They were pleasant, well-experienced miners. They knew what to do. He didn't have to teach them anything…but he constantly watched them.

He imagined the miners wearing little hats with lights on them. They had wheelbarrows and picks and shovels. In the beginning, the miners were marching from his healthy arm down into his smashed hand. They broke up the debris with their picks. They shoveled the debris into the wheelbarrows and carted it away, up into the arm, up to around the level of the elbow.

At some point, the tiny miners used hammers and new lumber, building new scaffolding and supports. They continued to march from his arm down into his hand and then back up his arm.

He observed them for three days, allowing no distractions.

By the end of three days, the smashed bits of bone in his hand had started repositioning themselves, moving back towards their original layout. The blood flow in the hand was healthy. No sign of gangrene. There was only severe weakness, soreness and achiness – the body's warning signs to be very careful.

After the first three days were over, he continued to do his visualizations now and then with the miners, but he also allowed himself to resume some of his other activities. Over time, the hand healed perfectly.

Case study: smashed fingers

Twenty years after learning about this technique, I shared the "tiny miners" method with a friend whose four fingers on his right hand were smashed by a falling boulder during a hiking accident. He was airlifted out.

The doctors wanted to amputate the fingers immediately.

My friend said no.

The doctors found what little skin they could from the ruptured fingers and wrapped it around the hash that had been his fingers' bones and muscles. Humoring him, they wrapped the "fingers" in gauze. Then they told him to come back in two days to have the fingers removed, to prevent gangrene from setting in.

Instead, he called me. I started him on the visualization with the little miners.

That same day, I started doing Yin Tui Na on his bandaged palm and the vicinity of his heart. My hands rested gently on the bloodied gauze or on his chest (I treated his chest / heart because he was in shock.)

As soon as the skin had regrown enough around his fingers, I also did Yin Tui Na, and eventually acupuncture, on them, as well. After a few weeks of *daily* treatment, with me doing FSR and him doing various visualizations for hours every day, I switched over to doing FSR only once a week, over the next few months. Every time I met with him, he assured me he was constantly filling the area with light, love, tiny miners, or whatever could hold his interest.

New blood vessels were the first tissues to regrow. His broken bones re-formed more slowly. Muscle and nerve function also returned. After several months, he had regained enough manual dexterity in his fingers that he was able to go back to his job as an acupuncturist.

Today, a casual observer would be hard put to notice the residual stiffness in two of his fingers.

You don't have to use miners. You can use anything that amuses you or fills you with love. The main thing to keep in mind is that something good is going into the injured or traumatized area and the debris is being moved out.

Over and over, something, anything, is lovingly going in and coming out of the injured area. This will keep your mind focused on the injured area. This will also help realign the electrical currents in the traumatized area, if they have been disrupted. These currents, when running correctly, carry instructions to the cells.

Most of the strongest rivers of current in the body run in fairly straight-ish lines, to and from the torso or head to the fingers and toes. The largest parts of the currents run in long straight-ish lines, parallel to the spine and the "straight-line" bones in the arms and legs, fingers and toes.

This technique of visualizing correct movement in and out of an injured area will not only restore the correct linearity to currents that, from injury or illness, have gotten swirly or are mistakenly running sideways or in whorls, it will also make the point to your brain that you do *not* want to be dissociated from this area.

The brain is not particularly clever. It doesn't know what is best for you. However, it is very, very obedient. If you repeatedly command your mind to do a particular thing over and over, your mind will quickly get good at doing it.

Practicing a new mental habit that you want to encourage can stop a previous, unhealthy mental habit, in favor of the new pattern. You don't necessarily need to get rid of the old dissociation habit or the negative thought pattern (unless, of course, you've given yourself a mental instruction to stay a certain way). Very often, you just need to actively work on the new, healthy pattern. This will change the way your brain works.

This ability to change a brain pattern is called neuroplasticity. "Neuroplasticity" is just a fancy way of saying "Your mind gets good at what it practices, whether you practice something healthy or unhealthy."

Ultimately, you alone are the boss of what your brain is practicing.

Summary

This chapter shared several methods for learning to mentally re-associate with an injury or dissociated area. The one I usually teach my patients is the first one: imagine highly focused light and energy – hold for a count of ten, relax, repeat, for a total of ten times of counting to ten.

In this method, your attention is focused very narrowly, like a laser. This is because you aren't actually trying to fix or heal the injured area: you are trying to pinpoint and alter the part of your *brain* that is saying, "We don't even *have* that body part."

Once the brain has been changed so that it says, "Huh. Look at that part of my body. Hey! It's injured." the mind can then give permission for the body to heal that spot. Healing will often kick in automatically.

The body is designed to heal.

The goal for treating dissociated areas is changing the way your brain is behaving: turning off your neural blockades by mentally focusing on the areas that had been walled off.

Then, you can resume active awareness of these areas. This will allow you to have the most efficient responses to your Yin Tui Na treatments.

Even when you have resumed awareness of an injured area by re-associating with it, both Yin Tui Na and the mental exercises can still be helpful to accelerate the healing.

Even a person who *doesn't* dissociate from his injuries and/or pain can still benefit by receiving supportive treatment such as FSR or some other light-touch therapy *and* by sending light and a tiny bit of energy to the injured or painful area.

Most people don't dissociate

Most of my patients presenting with injury or pain have *not* dissociated from their injuries. However, I still treat these patients with FSR, craniosacral, or other light-touch therapies, in order to hasten their healing and turn off their pain. I also teach most of them the light and energy exercises, in order to accelerate the healing and to prevent the formation of any dissociation mental behaviors.

If a patient *has* dissociated, I walk him/her through the light and energy technique while doing Yin Tui Na techniques on the injured area at the same time.

Then, *if* the flow of a patient's channel Qi is still disrupted after doing these protocols, I *might* do acupuncture to get the currents running correctly again.

Often, if the FSR treatment(s) have restored normal movement and vitality to the involved area *but* the electrical currents in the area haven't yet kicked in (this is rare), I will first try simply gently rubbing the area that had been disrupted in order to get the currents running correctly, if they aren't already. Almost always, no follow-up acupuncture needling is required.

Please, do not get too worried over when and how often you should do these mental re-association techniques. People with healthy, normal responses to pain and injury do something akin to these techniques automatically, even subconsciously.

These techniques are not rocket science. They are simple reminders of how humans are supposed to respond to pain or trauma, once the immediate crisis is over. These simple techniques to help you re-associate are provided here just in case you got yourself stuck in some dissociation mindset without even realizing you were doing it.

Finally, some people become extremely worried when they "see" that some part of their body is *dark*. Don't fall into this type of fear. Your body is *not* dark inside.

You aren't seeing what's actually in your body. You can't.

When you imagine that you are looking inside your body, you are picturing what your brain is willing to show you. If you see a dark place, it's because your brain is telling you that you are not allowed to see that place. In truth, the body part in question might be perfectly functional. Well, possibly it's injured and waiting to heal, and so it's not *perfectly* functional. But it's not actually dark inside.

The darkness in some body part is your brain's attempt at obeying your instruction to *pretend* to not *have* that body part.

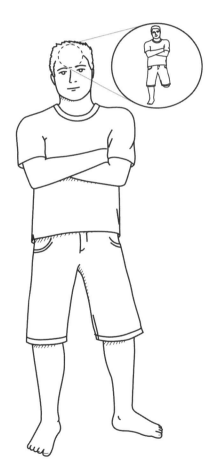

Fig. 5.1 The darkness you "see" in some body part is your brain's attempt at obeying your instruction to *pretend* to not *have* that body part. You actually *do* have that body part.

People with Parkinson's

Many people with Parkinson's are prone to ask *far* too many unnecessary questions about these techniques, such as wanting to know *exactly* how fast to count, or how many times or for how many minutes and under what *exact* circumstances they should do techniques for re-associating, or which body part should they address first, and so on.

Please, don't worry at all about the details. It truly doesn't matter if you are wearing jeans instead of sweat pants, or if the lights in the room are bright or dim or for that matter, which injuries you start with.

As an aside, a person who is inordinately worried about these types of details should consider that he might be stuck on pause mode rather than being merely dissociated from one or two body parts. Excessive wariness and constant risk assessment is characteristic of a person who has become stuck on pause. If you are stuck on pause, you should not be receiving hands-on therapy or trying to re-associate. Not yet, anyway.

If you are stuck in pause mode, whether or not you are also dissociated, do not use the techniques in this book until you have first turned off pause. Again, you can read about how to *diagnose* your own condition in Appendices I and II.

To *overcome* being stuck on pause, please read the book *Stuck on Pause*, referenced earlier in this chapter.

If you suspect you are *only* dissociated from some body part and are *not* stuck on pause, you can do one or more of the mental techniques in this chapter *and* allow yourself to be treated with Yin Tui Na.

After that, if the area is still painful or displaced tissues are still in need of restoration, do continue with the Yin Tui Na, but you don't *need* to do the exercises in this chapter. Then again, so long as any trace of injury, displacement, or pain remains, it can't hurt and might be helpful to do this chapter's "light and energy" exercise during your Yin Tui Na sessions, or any time you feel like it.

Again, the "light and energy" technique you will learn in this chapter can be used to accelerate healing even if there is *no* dissociation.

Chapter six

Turning off self-induced dissociation

Basic dissociation is a somewhat automatic process. A person has a bad experience or a nasty injury that he doesn't have time to deal with at the moment, and his subconscious mind just puts it aside, to be dealt with later.

Pathologies can arise when "later" never comes. The event or body part remains *stuck* in dissociation.

But sometimes, a person will *consciously* command himself, maybe several times, to not remember a specific event, or to not have pain in a specific body part.

This can lead to a situation in which the darkness-and-immobility in a given body part is well nigh impossible to get rid of without conscious work to first destroy the command. In cases of self-induced dissociation, in the response to the *basic* dissociation treatments described in the previous chapter, the dark area might re-appear following what seemed like, at first, a successful treatment, or it might even move to a slightly different location or become evasive – darting around in response to your attempts to focus on it.

Case study: I shall not feel my knee pain!

The previously mentioned patient with annoying knee pain remembered telling himself in college, "I don't want to have this knee pain. I *refuse* to notice it." He did this several times over two days, and it worked: his knee suddenly stopped hurting. He was able to resume his sports activities. He never had knee pain again…until he gradually, years later, slowly developed foot, ankle, leg and knee problems, "for no reason."

When I met him, he had *self-induced* a condition of dissociation in his right knee. His was not a case of automatically dissociating from knee pain during a crisis and forgetting to get around to dealing with the pain at a later time.

Fifteen years after self-inducing dissociation in his knee, when he came to see me for weakness and pain in his right ankle and feet, and even intermittent paralysis in his right knee, I asked him to imagine that he was looking around inside his right knee and lower leg. I asked him to view it as either filled with light or dark, whichever was easiest.

While looking around in his right-side leg, he "saw" that, as far as his imagination was concerned, his right leg, from just below the knee all the way down to the toes, was dark and immobile. In his mind's eye, the right *knee* didn't even *exist*.

He did the exercise of putting light and energy in his knee and holding it for a count of ten, and then repeating until he'd done ten sets of counting to ten. By the time he finished, the lower leg was filled with light. While he was doing this, I was doing FSR on his knee for what felt like, to me, a displaced knee cap.

About ten minutes later, mentally scanning his body again, he noticed that the darkness had returned. He attempted to put light in the center of the darkness again, but this time, the dark area kept moving around, sidestepping his attempts to focus on it.

That's when he laughingly told me what he'd mentally done to himself in college.

With self-induced dissociation situations, such as the above, you have to actually destroy the unhealthy mental command. If you don't, the problem might keep coming back or moving around indefinitely, trying to stay compliant with your still-active, self-created instruction.

State of mind matters

As it turns out, it's nearly impossible to *destroy* a negative instruction such as "don't acknowledge the pain" if you are in the same state of mind – you might say same degree of sympathetic ("fight or flight") mode – that you were in when you first *created* the instruction.

In order to destroy or supersede a previous fear- or pain-based instruction, you have to be in a more positive mindset than the mindset you used while creating the mental block. A mental command issued from a greater state of peace (parasympathetic mode) is able to counter or turn off a mental command issued while in a more negative (sympathetic) state of mind.[1]

To destroy a conscious (self-induced), fear-based command, you will need to first re-position your mind into what is sometimes called the "super-conscious mind" or "higher-conscious mind: a highly parasympathetic state. Some people call this part of the mind the intuitive mind or the heart-connected mind. It is a very circumspect, patient, loving, non-judgmental state of mind.

As an aside, the super-conscious mind is also considered to be the state of awareness that ideally might be attained by single-point meditation.

When one part of the "normal" mind – a blend of sympathetic and parasympathetic mode thoughts – is arguing with another sector of the normal mind, for example, over whether or not to quit smoking, or change some other stubborn habit, the battle can rage for years, with one side winning temporarily, and then the other side, always flipping back and forth, depending on one's mood or thoughts at the moment.

In eastern spiritual teachings, it is said that the *super*-conscious mind has the ability and the *authority* to immediately override and lastingly change the merely *conscious* mind, what you might call the "normal" mind.

---

[1] The word "sympathetic" in the case of sympathetic mode (fight or flight) does *not* mean sympathetic. This nomenclature was adopted in the 1800s, when the electric responses of nerves were discovered. The word "sympathetic" was used to describe nerves that activated muscles "in response" to an electric shock. The work "sympathetic" in this case meant "responsive." The (now archaic) medical use of the word "sympathetic" means "responds to electricity." This usage does *not* match up with our modern meaning of the word "sympathetic." In fact, it means quite the opposite.

I keep hoping that someone will change this outdated nomenclature.

An example: quitting smoking

A common example of this override is when a smoker, after decades of countless attempts at quitting smoking, suddenly has a moment of deep internal clarity and realizes, "I'm not a smoker anymore." And he never smokes again.

What has often happened in this situation is that a burst of awareness from the superconscious mind enabled him to see himself as a *non*-slave to the smoking habit. The smoker's-habit *brain pathways* that maintained a desire for and habit of smoking can then be instantaneously, permanently altered or destroyed.

Changing this habit usually has very little to do with slowly diminishing the effects of nicotine addiction. When a smoker, often unexpectedly, finds himself in a powerfully altered mental state, as if he is seeing himself "from a changed perspective," or "with greater and/or altered clarity" he finds he has spontaneously made the brain changes he's been long struggling to attain. Ask an ex-smoker for details.[1]

Technique for destroying self-induced dissociation

It's best to be relaxing in a quiet spot, sitting or lying down.

1. First, *define* the brain habit that you are going to get rid of.
For example, my patient in the above case study defined his habit as "ignoring my knee." He said this out loud a few times: "I have a habit of ignoring my knee." Then he said it mentally a few times.

By defining it, you will be able to simply use the words "the habit" while doing this technique, instead of going into a long verbal description, a long song and dance, during every repetition about what it is you are destroying.

2. Next, choose a short affirmation that resonates with you and confirms that you are part of something larger than yourself.

Examples of this affirmation are, "(Universal) Love and I are one." Or you might say, "I am part of the loving universe," "My heavenly Mother and I are one," "I am one with the Force," "I am one with Divine Spirit," or "My spiritual teacher/ guru/prophet and I are one" or "are connected."

3. Start silently saying your short, positive affirmation, one that confirms that your self, or your "soul" if you wish, is connected to some aspect of Universal Love.

Say it over and over. Focus on the words. Be so focused that your normal, always nattering mind stops its chatter and listens to what you are saying. Notice how your heart area feels. (If you are stuck on pause, you will probably not be able to notice how your heart area feels, and might even wonder what I mean by these words. This technique might not

---

[1] This profound, sudden change can occur with regard to many other types of brain habits as well. For example, the Jesuits (an education- and introspection-oriented monastic order within the Catholic church) have named this seemingly spontaneous brain alteration a "conversion experience." A conversion experience is a somewhat common event that can occur when a person powerfully turns his mind towards the greater perspective of an internalize sense of a higher power or suddenly sees himself as others see him, as opposed to constantly staying focused on his ego-based version of himself.

work for a person who is stuck on pause. A person on pause should first turn off pause. After that, he might not need to do this technique.)

As you say this affirmation for at least thirty seconds, or even several minutes, notice that, at some point, you start feeling calm.

That's good, but it's not good enough. Be pleased that you're feeling calm, but continue saying the affirmation.

At some point, a few seconds or a few minutes later, you will start feeling peace. Peace is a more dynamic feeling than mere calm. Peace allows the heart area to feel as if it is expanding, or even able to project its somatic (physical, in the body) *feelings* outward, into the universe. It's good that you are feeling peaceful, but that not's good enough. Be pleased that you are feeling peaceful, but continue saying the affirmation.

At some point, twenty seconds to ten minutes later, never wavering in your mental intensity, you will start feeling joy and a definite sense of relaxation and expansion in the heart area. Joy is expansive, radiant and, well, joyful. You will know when you are feeling joy.

Note: if you are stuck on pause, you might not be able to experience a feeling of joy because your mind is usually required to *avoid* feeling the sensations in the heart area and must instead stay focused on assessing whether or not you are at risk. Then again, *maybe* you might be able to. When a person uses *self-induced* pause, he might have the ability to go back and forth into either a personality that uses parasympathetic mode, (a personality who *can* feel joy) *or* into a personality that is uses pause. The ability to sometimes feel safe enough to be in parasympathetic mode can diminish or even cease if a blocker personality is created.

This rather complicated situation is discussed in detail in *Stuck on Pause*.

4. Once you get to joy, focus on the *feeling* of joy in the heart. Affirm, "This joy is my *real* self. This joy is what I *really* am.

Then, *use* this joyful personality. Your loving, joyful self speaks silently from the heart, sweetly and compassionately giving this command your brain: "Destroy the brain cells of that wrong habit." Or "Destroy the neural network of that wrong habit."

(The specialized nerve cells in the brain are called "neurons." The adjective form of the word is "neural.")

I read about this technique in a book on Eastern meditative science and yoga theory. The author, Paramahansa Yogananda, suggests that the joyful self use the phrase: "Cauterize the brain cells of this wrong habit."

"Cauterization" is medical burning, with exquisite precision, of cells that must be killed. He also suggests doing this brain-changing technique in the morning, when the mind and will power are freshest. [1]

---

[1] The information on this technique is in a book of short essays on yoga: *The Divine Romance*; Paramahansa Yogananda; published by Self-Realization Fellowship; second edition; 2000; p. 56. In this book, in essay #5, "What is Fate?", sub-heading, "How meditation changes your fate," the author discusses man's ability to make modifications in his brain, an ability that was considered impossible in the 1930s when these essays were written.

We now refer to this brain-altering ability as neuroplasticity. Most neuroplastic brain changes occur in response to changing our habits or our thought patterns.

Kill my own cells?!

Some people are taken aback at the idea of destroying their own neurons. Don't be. You have billions of neurons.

Think of it this way: if a few of them were cancerous would you hesitate to destroy them? No, you would cheerfully cauterize any cancerous brain cells.

These brain cell behaviors that you created in order to pretend you weren't hurt are, like cancer cells, *not* working in your best interest. You created these behaviors in a moment of emergency or in error. Now, it's time to get rid of them.

If neurons are creating mischief in your brain based on your own instructions, instructions that created blocker cells or re-routed existing cells into a blockade, it is reasonable to destroy them.

Think of it as cheerfully mopping up after spilling milk. It's *not* a big deal. Don't worry about the loss of a few misguided brain cells. We have billions, and don't even use *most* of the ones we have. Thanks to neuroplasticity, you'll be able to construct any new brain pattern you need.

A case study example

The first time I used this technique, I was disgusted at my years-long habit of falling asleep within a few minutes of sitting down for a long meditation.

After catching myself falling asleep, yet *again*, I performed this technique. I spent about five minutes getting calm, five minutes getting peaceful, and needed nearly ten minutes to build up a head of joy.

At some point, I realized I was overflowing with joy, so I stopped repeating the affirmation and joyfully commanded my brain to destroy "the habit."

I lovingly, joyfully commanded, over and over, "Cauterize the brain cells of this habit!" I imagined my heart had a little mouth on it, and was speaking upwards towards my brain.

After a few minutes, I felt an area of highly focused heat in one side of my head. At first, I considered being alarmed by this heat, but my heart, still joyful, assured me that I was OK.

Never again have I fallen asleep in meditation except for the times when I have been over-tired or over-fed. These few times were not sleeping from *habit*. They were due to my fatigue or physical grogginess.

This exercise is much more powerful that the techniques described in the previous chapter. Those techniques were for merely turning off automatic, "basic" dissociation. In those cases, the problem was that the brain had gotten stalled somewhere along the line of normal trauma processing and so wasn't able to move to the normal conclusion of "Now it's safe to process the trauma."

In those cases of automatic dissociation merely becoming suspended, the treatments described the previous chapter merely returns your attention to the place(s) in your body where the trauma was still waiting to "get to a safe place" so that it could be processed. Once processed, the body can resume the normal healing process that had been interrupted.

In the case of a *self-induced* mental habit of dissociation, the treatment has to be more powerful. You intentionally installed a wrong habit, a habit of evading a problem. Now, that habit is causing trouble. You need to destroy the wrong habit that you created.

More than one session might be needed

Please be aware, if the mental habit has been present for a long time or was self-induced, many, many repetitions of the technique might be necessary. Think of it as "chipping away" at a long standing pile of clutter.

The case I presented above, in which a habit of falling asleep during meditation was completely gone after one powerful session of self-instruction to "destroy the brain cells" of the wrong habit, is an example of a fairly simple habit change.

However, a *long-term* habit or self-instruction *might* need to undergo this technique in a short session every morning for weeks, or even longer, for as long as necessary, until the habit *and* the mental side effects of that habit are completely gone.

Also, after a few sessions, you may want to change your way of referring to your habit, or you may realize that the *actual* habit you want to get rid of is something else again. Fine. Change it up. Doing tidying up, doing house cleaning in your own mind, is a rewarding job. You can do it throughout your life.

What is this type of technique called?

You can refer to this type of self-healing as a type of yoga, in which you consciously bring some subconscious bad habit or fear-based mental behavior under the control of your peaceful consciousness or superconsciousness. (The word yoga means union, usually in reference to union of the soul with God. Yoga can also mean union of the soul with the mind – which is what you are doing when your joyful heart commands your brain to change. In the case of physical yoga exercises, the point is *feeling* the union of the mind and soul with the body.)

You can refer to this type of self-healing as mental medical Qi Gong (energy and mental-self control).

You can refer to this type of self-healing as "Cognitive Behavioral Therapy." This term just means consciously changing your mental behaviors. This type of powerful, effective therapy practiced by western psychologists since the 1980s has been rapidly replacing the "analysis" methods of psychological self-change that were based on outdated Freudian psychology.

It doesn't really matter what you call it. The main things to remember are:

You can change your brain habits.
No one else can do it for you.
You get to do it, cheerfully, and with a light heart, all by yourself.

Chapter seven

FSR technique: setting your hands on the patient

FSR is the most "Yin," the most subtle and non-invasive form of Tui Na. FSR technique can be broken down into four steps: 1) setting your hands on the patient, 2) following the patient's ensuing relaxation movements with your hands, 3) diagnostically making use of relaxation responses, if any, and 4) letting go.

This chapter and the three following chapters are devoted to these four steps.

Positioning the hands

With you and your practice partner sitting down, place the palm side of your hand flush against some part of the forearm of your partner. Then place your other hand on the opposite side of the forearm.

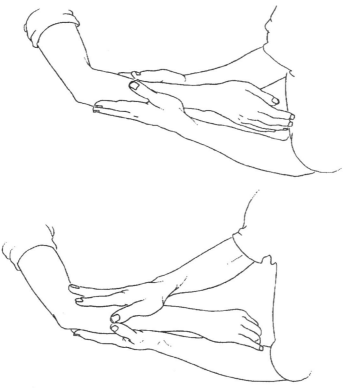

Fig. 7.1   Two examples of placing your hands on opposite sides of a body part

It does not matter exactly where your hands are. The important thing is that your two hands are more or less opposite each other.

Your own physical comfort is important. Position your chair so that you are comfortable.

If your patient or practice partner has an injury in the area you are holding, you may need to keep your hands fairly still for several minutes. If you are working on a Parkinson's patient, you may be sitting in one position, barely moving, for an hour. So your ability to get comfortable and stay relaxed is more important than the exact placement of your hands.

Slumping back in a soft chair may seem like a comfortable way to sit, but this type of "comfortable" is not easy to maintain for very long. You will be able to work longer and better if you can learn to sit upright, with good posture, while your arms suspend softly from the shoulders. Your wrists should be relaxed – able to move or flex in response to the patient's movements.

It's easiest for the beginner to practice FSR on a partner's arm. No physiological reason – it's just that arms are far easier to access: you can both be sitting in chairs when you work on arms. When you work on legs, the subject usually needs to be lying down.

Duration of treatment

I usually make one-hour appointments for working with a patient, and see patients once a week.

If you are doing FSR at home on a friend or loved one, the session can be whatever length of time is convenient for you. If fifteen minutes is the most time you have in a day, that's just fine. If you can do a little more, that's fine too.

More than an hour at a stretch can be draining for both of you. Remember, the patient is mentally working as well, putting light and energy into the area you are working on.

It is fine to do FSR every day, every other day, or once a week. The main thing is you don't want to stress the patient or put pressure on him to "hurry up and heal!"

Asking permission

Before grabbing your patient's or your practice partner's arm or leg, ask permission to hold the arm or leg.

After getting comfortably settled into your work chair or stool, with the patient sitting in a chair or lying down on the treatment table with his shoes off, ask, "May I hold your arm?" or "May I hold your leg?"

Ask permission every time you begin to work on a patient. This simple question becomes rather ceremonial. It is a very polite way of honoring the patient's autonomy. You aren't just going to hold fire until your patient looks comfortable and then grab for his arm or leg. You ask permission to hold, and then after the patient says, "Yes," you start.

This may seem very formal and unnecessary, but you will see very quickly that patients learn to anticipate this little bit of courtesy and respond pleasantly.

Of course, the first time you work on a patient and ask this, they may reply, "Of course! That's what I'm here for!" But after a few sessions, they will understand that they are participating in a respectful ceremony.

Use your palms

The firm support and *contact* over the widest possible area is the main thing

Usually, the *palms* of your hands are the main contact points. Do *not* try to hold the patient with your fingers. Your fingers can of course be making contact, as well, but the center of the strength of your holding comes from the palms of your hands.

When we hold something with our fingers, our fingers curve inward (flexed), which is to say, with the fingers moving towards the "fist" position. Notice in the illustrations that opened this chapter, in Fig. 7.1, how the fingers are the opposite of flexed – they are slightly extended. In terms of muscle movements, "extended" means the opposite direction of "flexed." This finger extension is not always necessary, but sometimes, depending on the curve of the patient's skin, the fingers need to be relaxed enough that they assume either an extended or flexed position in order to get the center of the palm of the hand firmly connected to the patient.

Of course, there will be times when the palm of the hand doesn't fit easily. For example, when holding the arch of the foot, you will place one hand over the top of the foot – directly over the arch area (the "saddle" of the foot) – and the other hand on the sole of the foot, *under* the arch. But, if the size and angles of the arch prevent the *palm* of your hand from getting solid, flat contact on the sole of the arch, you might use the *back* of your hand, or even the backs of your fingers, instead of the palm of your hand, to provide firm support to the sole of the foot in the arch area.

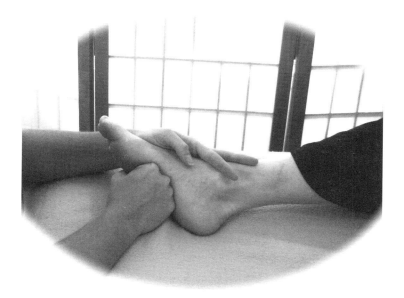

Fig. 7.2   Using the back of the hand to make firm contact with the sole of the foot

You should *not* grip with your fingers just because you're working on an area that is hard to access with your palm; you should find some way to make firm contact with some part of your hand that will create the sensation that the patient's body is being held in place with an ace bandage (also known as an elastic bandage) – but *not* held in place with vice grips.

Again, the firm support and *contact* over the widest possible area is the main thing – *not* the electrical properties contained in the palm of your hand.

Pressure

The amount of pressure that your hands exert on the practice partner is *very important*. You should make firm, fairly complete contact even if there is clothing in between your hands. You want to create the sensation of firm contact over as large an area as possible. Your hands are like a snug blanket. The goal is to hold your practice partner with such complete support that, very soon, he doesn't notice your motionless hands.

Because the sensation of support is more important than the exact, precise location of where you are holding, it is important that you find a way to nestle your hands into the contours of your partner's body part, even if such a holding position is not exactly the location of holding that you originally had in mind. Sometimes, when you have gotten your hands nestled into a place that feels comfy and "settled in," your practice partner might even volunteer that you have put your hands in "just the right place" even though he didn't know there was any place that particularly wanted to be held.

Now let's back up a bit and look more closely at what you are doing, looking at one hand at a time. Let's assume in the following explanation that you are putting one hand on the upper side of your partner's forearm, and your other hand underneath his arm. In actual practice, of course, one hand might be on the left side and the other on the right side. But for clarity, let's assume that your hands are on the "top" (closer to the ceiling) and "bottom" (closer to the floor) of the partner's forearm.

Upper hand

If you are sitting in a comfortable position, you will be able to let your upper hand drop gently from your shoulder and come to rest on the partner. Your hand should be resting like a dead weight, with the full weight of your hand plopped down on your partner. Now, add just a bit *more* pressure – enough so that your partner's skin isn't possibly going to slip out from under your hand. You should be using a fair amount of force, by the way. If you are using *any* muscles to *prevent* your hand from pushing too hard onto your partner, you are holding too lightly. Use gravity, and then a bit more.

If you aren't sure what I mean by "dead weight" and then a little more, you might want to abandon your partner for a moment and try this practice exercise: sit in an armless chair. Let your hand flop down onto your thigh. Let your hand just sit there, held in place by gravity. Notice that your hand isn't making *complete* contact with your leg: there's a gap on the palm of the hand where air is present. Now, leave your hand in place and lean forward just a few inches so that your hand is supporting the weight of your torso. Notice that your hand is now making firm contact with your leg. It's not that you are trying to push *against* your leg. It's more that the weight of your torso is causing your hand to make a very *complete* contact with your leg. The force needed to make a complete contact is the exact right amount of pressure to use in FSR.

Again, *don't* push your hand hard into your thigh as if you were trying to leave an imprint of your hand: that would be too much pressure. Don't rest your hand gingerly, as if your thighs were sunburned: that would be not enough pressure. Let your shoulders relax and sag down. Let your hand rest heavily on your thigh while supporting your slightly forward body. That is the exact correct amount of pressure for your top hand. Now, take this hand off your thigh and respectfully allow it to plop back down with the same degree of weight onto your practice partner's arm.

Lower hand

Use the exact same amount of pressure with the lower hand that you use with the upper hand.

If you want, you can abandon your partner again for a moment and practice holding your thigh again, but this time you will use both hands. Let your first hand flop down onto one side of your thigh, and place your other hand on the opposite side of your thigh. Lean your torso forward just a bit so that the hands must make a more complete contact in order to stay where they are.

Another image: imagine that your thigh is a mound of bread dough. Use as much pressure between the hands as you would need to use to keep the lifeless bread dough from dropping to the ground. Do not hold the limp "bread dough" gingerly and do not hold it with your fingertips. You might even spread your fingers apart so that you can get the centers of your palms as close to the "bread dough" as possible. The fingers might be slightly flexed or slightly extended – whatever position best enables you to have the palms of your hands as firmly connecting to the thigh as possible. Have a firm grip on the two sides of the "bread dough" of your thigh, but don't be leaving imprints of your hands or fingers in your flesh. Just hold it enough so that even if the thigh goes completely limp, it won't fall to the floor.

The point that your hands need to be making to your partner is this: even if your muscles in this area were to become as limp as bread dough, I am giving you enough support so that you won't fall to the floor.

Your hands are saying, "I've got you, you are safe, you may become as limp as you want, and no harm will come to you."

Try placing both hands on your partner's forearm again, using the same amount of support that you used to support your thigh when you imagined it was as limp as bread dough.

Always use two hands

When your hands are on either side of the partner's body part, your two hands should be pressing on *each other* with the necessary amount of force.

You *never* press down on the partner's body part with just one hand. If you do this, the partner will reflexively use energy to push back against your hand. When you are "holding" your partner between your two hands, the pressure you are using is NOT pressure being applied to the partner – your two hands are applying equal pressure against *each other*. By supporting the partner with *two* hands, and the two hands are pressing against *each other*, your partner doesn't need to "push back" against anything. Your partner is being supported. The two hands are pushing firmly on *each other*, not on your partner.

Again, when you are holding your partner, what you should really be doing is pressing your hands together. It just so happens that a partner's body part is in between your hands. Ignore the partner's body part. If you want to focus on anything, focus on how your two hands are pressing on each other even though something has come between them.

When your focus is on your two hands applying firm pressure on each other, and you are ignoring the body part that is resting between your hands, you will be feeling what it's like to provide firm, supportive holding.

Eventually, you will be able to notice all sorts of things going on in the partner's body part, while keeping your primary focus on your own hands.

You will then be able to notice subtle changes or tensions in your partner's body part, and you can then use this information to modify the exact placement of your hands, or the exact amount of pressure that you are using, so as to help the partner relax even more. These modifications will be almost automatic, even reflexive. They will occur in response to what your partner's body is silently telling you. Don't worry about what your hands will do at this point – soon enough, they will be working with your partner on their own, without your mind getting involved.

Much as a good dairy farmer intuitively knows how to touch each of his cows to keep them calm, at some point your *hands* will know just how much pressure to use in response to each of your partner's body's signals, even if you don't consciously know how much pressure is needed.

How much pressure to use – yet again

"How much pressure?" is *the* most frequently asked question.

I repeat, you should use as much force as you need to make your practice partner feel perfectly supported. If the effect of gravity should suddenly stop working on your partner's body part, your pressure would continue to hold the partner in the same place.

All of us maintain a certain amount of unconscious pressure in our muscles – at least enough to combat gravity.

If you are holding with at least the force of gravity, the partner will be able to stop unconsciously fighting the force of gravity in that particular body part. This unconscious work of combating gravity (on the part of the partner) can cease. The part of the partner's body that you are holding can relax much more deeply than usual.

Oddly enough, when you provide enough support, supplanting all the tension the partner was maintaining to combat gravity and to support his anticipation of needing to move in self-protection, the partner's body soon will be *unable* to tell that you are applying any force at all. The partner will feel as if, for all intents and purposes, your hands are not even there.

Have you ever swaddled a crying baby? Swaddling blankets are wrapped so snugly around a baby that he can't even move – not at all. And when the baby is swaddled snugly enough, he is able to relax. When he is so constrained by the tight blanket that he *can't* move his own muscles, when he doesn't *need* to move his own muscles to combat the strange, heavy world that is such a contrast to his previous, weightless world in utero, he relaxes as if he was once again floating and weightless.

When ranchers need to calm a frantic calf, they usher him into a "squeezer," or "press," a simple device consisting of boards on both flanks of the calf. A rope pulls the two sides of the press together, squeezing the calf until he can't move. When the calf feels sufficient support, he relaxes. His muscles, being supported by the press, don't need to maintain any tension of their own. The calf calms down both physically and mentally.

The principles of swaddling and pressing are the same principles used in Yin Tui Na: solid, firm support applied to a patient in a particular body area can physically and mentally relax that body area.

Don't be "gentle"

Do not hold gently; nothing can be more annoying. Resting your hands or fingertips ever so lightly on a partner is a sure way to either tickle or irritate him.

Hold the body part with such support that even if the table on which your partner's body is resting was to be pulled away, your holding would prevent his body from falling to the floor.

Don't manipulate

Don't try to physically *or even mentally* manipulate the limb you are holding. At this stage, when you are practicing how to hold without either insufficient or excessive physical or mental pressure, consider that any intention on your part, even for the good of the patient, is a form of psychological manipulation. So don't be imagining any particular outcome as a result of your support. Have *no* intention in mind for how the practice partner should respond.

Pressure without intention: the harried parent example

The following example illustrates what I mean by solid support without intention.

Picture the scene: a harried mother (or father, of course) is trying to cook dinner. She is standing at the stove, stirring food in two pots. One pot has almost come to a boil and needs to be watched closely. The other pot is bubbling away and needs frequent stirring. Just out of arm's reach, her four-year old child is pestering her two-year old child. The younger child is starting to scream in frustration. The mother cannot reach them because she is stirring the dinner, plus she is talking to her friend on the phone; the phone is the old fashioned kind, attached by a cord to the wall.

She is not using her hand to hold the phone, the phone is cradled between her ear and her raised shoulder. She is alternating between telling the youngsters to stop fighting and trying to arrange a babysitting swap with her friend for tomorrow.

Meanwhile, she is also holding a baby on her hip. It is not her *own* baby; she is babysitting for another neighbor, who should be home shortly. The mother has the neighbor's baby wedged up against her left hip and she has her left arm wrapped around the baby. Baby is stuck between the firm left hip and the snug left arm. Baby is in *solid*. Baby is going *nowhere*.

With her right arm, mother is now alternating between adding some spice to the dinner and tasting it. Mother is still listening to her friend on the phone and is stage-whispering to the older child a command to stop hitting the younger child with the stuffed weasel.

Here is my question: who is the most contented person in the room?

If you guessed the neighbor's baby, you are absolutely right. The baby is looking around, taking it all in, reveling in the fact that he doesn't have any social interactions going on. Baby is being held so closely that he can't move. With this level of firm support, baby doesn't even notice that he is being held. Baby has such complete trust in that firm support coming from the hip and the embracing arm that baby does not notice the pressure from the mother's hip and arm. Also, and most importantly, *the mother is not paying any attention to the baby* with her eyes or words. The baby is physically relaxed and comfortable.

Of course, when the baby's mother returns, baby will probably go into its regular routine of crying or cooing at its own mother, doing all the things he has already learned to do to fulfill its mother's expectations. But while the baby is being held snugly, tightly on the busy mother's hip with no one looking at him, no one cooing at him, no one expecting anything of him, being *completely ignored*, he is able to take it all in with wide-eyed wonder, amusement or contentment, and his body is physically at peace.

How is the above mother holding the baby? Snugly! Firmly! That's the way you hold a person with an unhealed injury.

The biggest mistake that therapists make in the beginning is that they give support to their patients as if the patients were their *own* babies: cooing over them, worrying over them. You should hold a person with an unhealing injury as if you are busy with thinking of something else and your are holding *someone else's* baby: a baby that you don't need to emotionally interact with.

Comfort for the practitioner

In the example above, the mother is doing whatever she needs to do to be comfortable. No doubt she has one hip swung way out to the side to support the baby. This isn't an example of "good posture," but by having one hip out to the side as a seat for the baby, the mother is able to be very comfortable while holding that extra weight.

What with gravity, the mother's hip, *and* the additional, very firm lateral support provided by the left arm, the baby is nice and snug.

The amount of pressure you should use is the same as the mother is using on the baby: enough so that the baby can breathe easily, but can't really move around too much.

This amount of pressure should be comfortable for you. If you find that you are getting tired arms or sore hands, possibly you are using too much pressure or your chair is not at the right height. If you are not relaxed, it will be hard to give perfect support to your patient.

Comfortable pressure becomes imperceptible

We can quickly become used to external forces pushing or resting on the skin. When we wear clothes and shoes to which we have become accustomed, we no longer notice them. Within a few moments of putting on a comfy pair of old shoes, we have no awareness of the shoes pressing against our feet.

When we wrap on an ace bandage over a weakened, sprained area, we quickly forget that the bandage is there: we very quickly stop perceiving the force of the bandage, but we move better because, deep inside, we know that bandaged area is being supported.

One excellent FSR practitioner that I know says that, when he sits for an hour not moving, with his hands cradling a wounded foot, he feels like a human cast. That's a very good analogy. Of course, a plaster of Paris cast or a more modern plastic cast gives solid support, but it is rigid, cold and cannot conform perfectly to the changing contours of a live human. A "cast" made of human hands gives a far better level of support: it is warm and conforms more perfectly to the skin of the patient.

Practice time!

Ask permission to support whatever area you are going to hold.

Place your hands on your practice partner's forearm or leg and experiment with positioning your hands until you find a pose that is very comfortable for you.

Have your partner tell you if your hands feel too pushy, too light, or if they feel just right.

Have your partner then try the same on you.

Take turns seeing how it feels to hold someone's forearm. If you think you are comfortable with the forearm, try holding the upper arm. Try holding the partner's thigh or lower leg. Play with this. See what it feels like to hold supportively but without expectation, and how it feels to be held.

Above all, notice that, sometimes, especially as you get faster and more relaxed about putting firm pressure on right from the start, the practice partner's muscles will almost instantly respond by relaxing or moving a bit, or sometimes moving a lot, in the area where you are holding.

As you get more familiar with this type of holding, try pretending that your confidence level has increased to the point that, as soon as you set your hands on your practice partner, you are instantly applying just the right amount of pressure. In other words, you *don't* want to get in the habit of spending five minutes figuring out exactly how much pressure to use. Have confidence.

Practice resting your hands firmly and opposite to each other until you get to the point that you know, even before you set your hands on your partner, just how much pressure you will be wanting to use. From the moment you start to place your hands on your partner, do it confidently.

Working through clothes

As mentioned, this technique can be practiced on a partner's clothed limbs. At the very beginning, it may be easier for your *mind* to accept the fact that you can feel a partner's response if you are working with bare skin, so you might want to work on a partner's bared arm, to start.

As soon as you feel ready, work on clothed areas, as well, in order to increase your confidence.

Review

Though I'm being blatantly redundant here, I repeat that touching, if done too lightly, is an irritant. Oppositely, when touching is done with too *much* pressure, so that it causes pain, it may even generate a pulling-away response. If there is one-sided pressure, as opposed to two-handed pressure, the subject cannot help but push back, instead of relaxing.

The type of touching used in FSR is the confident, *firm* gentleness with which a mother holds someone else's child while she's ignoring it by being mentally occupied with something else. FSR requires supportive contact that does not impose a command, but conveys non-judgmental stability and safety.

"Forceless" touch

Most often, the beginner is far too delicate, employing an irritating, "gentle" touch. The problem is that he is trying to be "forceless." The pracitioner isn't supposed to be "forceless."

The word "forceless" in the name Forceless, Spontaneous Release applies to the *perception* of the *patient*, not to the amount of pressure used by the practitioner. It also applies to the *intention* of the practitioner, inasmuch as the practitioner isn't using any directional force on the patient, but is just sitting there pressing his own hands against *each other*, and not thinking that he's applying force to the *patient*, per se.

The more pressure you use, to a point, the less the patient will notice it. When the patient perceives no directional, instructional force coming from your hands, and instead only perceives that he is being firmly supported, little movements in his muscles will manifest. These movements are spontaneous relaxations in response to this support.

Many, many times a health practitioner has come to visit my office, bringing along his patient, in order to see if he is doing FSR correctly. Within seconds of me setting my hands on the patient, the patient says to his practitioner, "Janice is using *way* more pressure than you do! *Way* more."

Use plenty of pressure. Unless your patient complains, or you are leaving indentations in your patient's skin, you are probably *not* using too much pressure.

You are using some firm force, pressing your hands against each other and paying not much attention to whatever's in between them.

Your *patient*, very soon, doesn't notice it. To your *patient's* perception, the treatment is forceless.

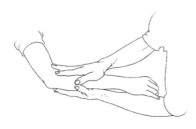

Chapter eight

FSR technique part II: following the movement

The relaxation response

When you practice holding your practice partner's forearm, you will notice, eventually, that at the moment when you place your hands on your partner using firm support, an *immediate or fairly rapid* and, sometimes, visually perceptible change occurs in the position of those muscles in your partner which are immediately under your point of contact.

This movement arises from the immediate, localized relaxation of the partner's body part in response to your support. The change may even be *visually* perceptible to you and/or your partner because your hands, making firm contact, will perceptibly move even as your partner's forearm relaxes. The movements might be subtle or glaringly obvious. If subtle, so that you can't see the movement in the *partner's* arm, you *might* nevertheless notice that *your* hand positions have been immediately altered ever so slightly from the exact position in which you started.

Because of your commitment to supportive contact on your partner's skin, when his skin/underlying muscles move, your hands move along with him. If you notice that your hands are resting in a slightly different position than they were when they were very first placed on the partner's arm, then you can be assured that this is because the partner's muscles and skin have moved.

If your partner's skin moves, keep holding: follow the movement. Maintain contact, and let your hands be carried to a new position by the movement.

Types of relaxation movement

Often, the relaxation response is small and gentle.

Sometimes, the relaxation response is a bit jerky.

Other times, the relaxation response will actually move back and forth, instead of being a simple, one-way move. Fine. Keep your hands in place while the area being held moves back and forth.

Now and then, the relaxation might even feel as if circular movement is occurring in the skin under your hands, or in the fascia that's just under the skin that's under your hands. You may feel as if one or both of your hands needs to move in a circle in order to adhere to the skin or fascia's movement.

It's actually impossible for your hand to move in complete circles while maintaining contact, so what you'll do is let your hand rotate a bit, maybe as much as forty-five degrees, following the movement. Then, when you've rotated at the wrist as many degrees as you can comfortably tolerate, quickly pull your hand off the skin and bring it back to a comfortable wrist position. Set your hand back down on the partner – and let it continue following the rotation, if any, in the partner. If the partner's fascia feels as if it's doing a lot of "unwinding," you may need to pull your rotated hand off and quickly set it back down a dozen times, or more, to provide the illusion of constant support on your partner without making a corkscrew out of your wrist.

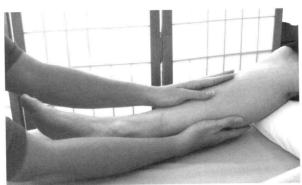

Fig. 8.1
These two pictures are the first and last of a continuous photo group, with the camera mounted on a tripod. The camera started when the hands were placed on the partner. The photo group ended after two seconds, when the partner's skin stopped moving.

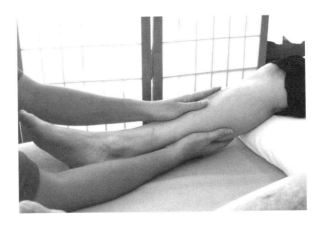

Fig. 8.2
Notice in the second photo the very slight tilt in the wrist muscles of the practitioner's upper hand. The third finger is no longer visible. In the lower hand, the index finger is no longer visible: it has rotated away from the camera. The arm just above the wrist has elongated slightly.

A question

You might ask, "What if my partner is already relaxed? If so, he cannot relax in response to being held." Don't worry. If your partner is fighting gravity, he is doing work

46

and, therefore, is not perfectly relaxed. One can safely assume that all *healthy* patients/partners are not in a state of perfect relaxation and *will* relax somewhat in response to being supported.

When your hands are applied to his forearm (or any body part), your hands will supplant some of the partner's inherent tension; the touched area will relax its share of internal muscular grip accordingly. This small release of muscle tension will create a movement in the skin and underlying muscles, such that the practitioner's hands will find themselves resting on the partner in a slightly different position than when they began.

This change might not be perceptible to the receiving practice partner if he has his eyes closed. Because he *felt* no vector of force being applied, the partner will most likely think that nothing has happened except that he briefly felt the initial contact from your hands. If the partner *sees* that your hands have moved slightly in the first moment after you placed your hands on him, he will most likely assume that *you* have initiated some movement: *you* were moving your hands around.

This may seem redundant, but here goes: even if *you* feel a significant relaxation in your practice partner's arm so that your hands move a tiny bit or even a good quarter of an inch or more, if your partner's eyes are closed during the time of contact and subsequent movement, *he* might not detect that anything has happened at all other than the fact that you are supporting his arm. If he *does* notice that his muscles have moved, he may very well accuse *you* of having moved them. Because he did not give any conscious movement command to his muscles, it may be hard for the patient/partner to realize that his muscles moved reflexively of their own accord. It is very common for students, working on each other, to accuse the "practitioner" half of the pairing of having imposed the movements that occur in the area in question.

The patient's sense of what's happening

Sometimes, though not often, the practice partner might say something like, "My muscle movement wasn't reflexive: I was *consciously* doing that. I felt that I had a choice as to whether to move, or not."

This description of the inner conflict, or choice, can be a correct understanding, in some cases. The body might have been somewhat reluctant to move, and yet wanted to move. Healthy relaxation occurs when the person allows himself to move in the manner that the area seems to "want."

Consider this: when you firmly hold a startled, panicked child until he calms down, that child does not perceive that you have done anything to him. And yet, he calms down quickly if you hold him firmly enough, with enough confidence. So you *have* done something, and you can feel him relax in your arms as a result. But he won't have *felt* that you've done anything. Not only that, the child may be aware that he *made a choice* when he relaxed: he *could* have stayed upset, but he chose to relax. But actually, he was more easily *able* to relax because of the support that he was getting.

Sometimes, when people see me, as teacher, demonstrate this technique on their partner, they want to protest that the partner's arm movement was not due to relaxation on the part of the partner. They accuse me: "You were shoving their arm around!" I have to insist that I was doing nothing of the kind.

Other students take the opposite stand: "Nothing happened in *response* to your hands, the partner just *happened* to relax a little at the same time you put your hands on him."

Well, of course. That's the whole point: the partner will relax when supportive hands are placed on his skin. This relaxation *can* be extremely fast and it may seem to the person being held as if nothing significant has actually happened.

Because the response is so unpredictable, sometimes hard to feel on the part of the partner and so startling to the new practitioner, it is possible that both the practitioner and the partner may want to insist that the *other* person must have been intentionally "moving the forearm around."

Don't try to think it through too much. Just practice holding someone and observe what happens.

How many sessions will be needed?

Sometimes enough relaxation can occur in response to this type of *brief* holding that a significant release of tension or repositioning of displaced bone or tissue will occur. Sometimes – and this is the point – in response to this supportive touch, relaxation and awareness of the area can increase in an area that previously, due to tension or dissociation, was resistant to *healing*.

Then again, sometimes it takes longer to get a response. In people who have dissociated from a body part or who haven't yet healed from some trauma, it might take a long, long time, even weeks or months of once-a-week, one-hour treatments, in order to get a response. Then again, if your patient does the mental work in chapter five, or chapter six, if needed, the responses almost always come much more quickly – sometimes even in the first session.

Then again, I had one patient with forty-year old (since childhood) neck vertebral displacements. She was dissociated *and* was using self-induced pause. When we started doing work together, little signs would pop up in her head, in her imagination, with lettering spelling out: "Don't let anyone work on you! Go hide in the cave! (Her mental image of the inside of her head, when she was finally brave enough to imagine looking there, was a cave surrounded by barbed wire.)

Slowly, over a long time, we figured out that she needed to do the mental exercises for self-induced pause, for dissociation, and for self-induced dissociation. Even so, after doing all this, she still needed more than a *year* of weekly craniosacral treatments and FSR on her neck, back, and shoulders before she felt deeply at peace inside. Unexpectedly, after she'd been feeling peaceful inside for over a year, her neck bones suddenly all slid back into place while I was holding her neck. Instantly, she could once again turn her neck from side to side for the first time in decades. I am certain that any method that used *any* amount of force would never have been able to get through to her. I share this rare case study to drive home the point that some people need more time than others.

But *most* people, if they do the mental exercises for getting rid of whatever is inhibiting healing, be it dissociation, self-induced dissociation, pause, or all three will respond fairly quickly to FSR once the mental blocks are gone.

Still, no two people are the same.

Maintain the support during movement

Holding on, keeping the hands in supportive contact even while the person responds with a small tiny movement or by more obvious moving around, is a critical part of the support. When you hold a person with supportive touch, you are rather implying that you are there for him, holding him for as long as needs be. This means that, if your patient's arm (or whatever body part) does move in response to being held, you have an unspoken obligation to continue to follow the movement wherever it goes, providing support until you receive a "let go" signal. This signal is discussed in the next chapter.

Sometimes this means that a practitioner's hands may end up in a *very* different position than where he started. But wherever the patient goes, there you, the practitioner, *must* follow.

Letting go temporarily, moving to a more comfortable position

If, in response to your support, the partner's arm (or body part) moves in such a direction that you can no longer hold on comfortably or keep your balance, then, of course, you should let go and smoothly, quickly, reposition your hands in a way that will allow you to be comfortable while continuing to provide support.

The partner will not go to pieces if you let go for a quick moment.

Sometimes, if you sense that the partner's body truly does not want you to let go, but you simply must move to a more comfortable position, then rotate your arms around or move your torso in such a way as to accommodate to the new holding position without actually lifting your hands off the skin, if possible. As soon as the partner's body part stops moving and is getting settled in in the new position, you can smoothly and quickly lift your hands off and resettle them in a more comfy position.

Use your common sense with this; there is no value in having the practitioner get a crick in his neck. Picture a worried child wanting to be held tightly by a parent: the parent can move as much as he needs to get himself in a comfortable position and the child will not fall apart while the parent does so. However, once the parent gets to a position of maximum comfort and stops fidgeting, the child also settles down more deeply.

A common mistake that students make is that they assume the response will not occur for several seconds. Students often ignore that first, instantaneous "flinching" movement, and settle in to watch for something dramatic.

The tiny "flinch" may well be the reflexive relaxation response you are looking for.

Sudden jerks

The practitioner must be prepared to hold on during those rare response movements that are large or jerky. If your hands are committed to supporting your patient and suddenly the patient's arm (or whatever) twists or bounces, you need to hang on even though you may feel, for a split second, as if you are being carried somewhere unexpected.

The warning signal

As you become more experienced with this technique, you may begin to notice that a faint electrical discharge that feels sort of like static energy moving through your own hands and even up your arms will often precede a major jerk or twist on the part of the patient. If you are in tune with this sort of thing, you can use these static discharges as a warning to brace your feet on the floor or loosen up your elbows in preparation for a sudden lurch or lunge.

An anecdote

I was holding onto a patient's thigh and getting no response at all. She'd been numb in that leg following a bad bicycling accident. I was standing at the side of the treatment table, mentally settling in to a comfortable daydream. My hands were holding firmly on her left thigh but my mind was rapidly moving to a place a thousand miles away.

After about ten minutes, I felt a flash of static electricity in my arms, but before I could even steady myself in response, I found myself lying across her legs, my head hanging down the opposite side of the table from where I'd been standing a moment earlier. My hands were still gripping firmly on her thigh, which had rotated medially so abruptly that the force of the rotation had lifted me off my feet and flung me towards the opposite side of the table.

She laughed. She had felt nothing at all in her leg even while she saw me sailing through the air, over her legs. A moment later, she sighed with relaxation and announced that she had feeling in her leg.

This *extreme* tossing around has only happened to me once. But many times a patient's head, arm, leg, or foot has shaken me like a terrier shaking a rat.

You never can know just what's going to happen. So tell your hands to hang on, and tell your mind to relax and mind its own business.

This simple holding and the almost immediate response (in uninjured areas) that you can notice by movement occurring under your hands are the basic events of FSR. Practice it on someone else. It is very hard to practice it on yourself.

Doing FSR on yourself

Then again, I received an email from a person with Parkinson's, whose diagnosis had been confirmed by three different doctors, who had moved to "the middle of nowhere," to care for her aged, ailing father. There was no one around to help her, so she did FSR on herself.

She wrote that sitting on the sofa in the evenings after her father went to bed, she held her long-injured foot. Sometimes, she placed her hands over her heart, to comfort herself. She found herself enjoying the therapy. She wrote that doing FSR on herself changed her ability to notice how her body was *feeling*.

She recovered from Parkinson's disease, and used no physical therapy other than the holding provided by her own hands.

Of course, it's far easier to have someone do this for you. But anything is possible. Everyone's different.

An old, forgotten injury on your healthy practice partner

If your "healthy" practice partner's arm does not respond in any way, if there is *no* relaxation response, it is very possible that the partner has an old injury in the arm you are holding. If so, use the other arm. If the other arm also does not respond, try having the partner lie down and work on the partner's calves.

When I've taught classes in this technique, there's usually one person out of the twelve students whose body part doesn't relax as predicted. A quick verbal interview usually uncovers a medical history of broken bone or injury in the area that didn't relax in response to being held.

In the classes I teach, every once in a great while, maybe once every few years, a practice partner will turn out to be stuck on pause or dissociated. He is *not* going to be able to have a relaxation response. If your practice partner doesn't seem to respond, try working with a few other people.

So when choosing a practice partner, you might *not* want to work, at first, with someone with a history of many broken bones and/or a "high tolerance for pain." A high tolerance for pain is often an indication that a person has become very good at dissociating from pain or is even using pause mode.

Again, if your partner doesn't respond, at all, to your holding, don't worry, don't assume that you are doing something wrong. The unresponsive partner may well have an old injury in the area(s) in question *and* might not even remember the old injury. But do consider working on someone else, if you don't get any responses with your first practice partner. If you can work on several people, that would be best.

Don't be shy about recruiting practice partners from among your friends; most people don't mind having their arm held for a few minutes. If someone does mind, or feels uneasy about it, that person may well have some unhealed injury or history of trauma in the arm and might not consciously be aware of it.

Never force yourself on someone who does *not* want to be touched.

Having said that, I've observed that *most* people quickly learn to enjoy and appreciate this supportive therapy.

Chapter nine

FSR technique: letting go

Now that you know to keep holding on to your patient no matter where or how much his skin and muscles move around or don't move around, you need to learn when to let go. The rule is: let go when the patient's skin tells you to let go.

A person's skin in the area where you are holding will perform what feels like an electric-charge reversal when your support is no longer wanted. If you keep holding when the support is no longer wanted, the person's skin will start sending you an electrical message that pushes you away, ever so slightly, breaking your skin contact. This is a "Let go" signal.

To improve your awareness of these small but distinct Let go signals, you may want to practice the steps below.

The "Let go" signal

Ask permission to hold some body area. Hold that area. This time, while following with your hands the movement of the practice partner's skin as he relaxes, notice that there has been a tiny, momentary sensation of magnetic pull or "connectedness" between your hands and the skin of the partner. This sensation can be felt even if clothing is between your hands and the partner's skin.

The sensation might be described as feeling magnetically bonded, or "pulled in" to your practice partner's skin. A moment later, or maybe as long as ten minutes, or even an hour, later, you will notice that your skin ceases to feel bonded to your partner's skin: the magnetic bond seems to be broken.

In fact, your hand may detect the opposite sensation: it may seem as if your partner's skin is pushing your hand away ever so slightly. You'll notice that, without your realizing it, your hand has slightly lifted itself off the skin or clothing of your practice partner. This is the signal to Let go.

The Let go sensation is similar to the sensation of trying to put two similar magnet ends together. The force that repels the north end of one magnet from the north end of another magnet is very much like the force that a person's skin exerts on the hands of someone who has been holding on for long enough.

Going back to the first feeling, the feeling of being magnetically attached, this sensation of magnetic connection has been compared to the feeling that exists between two socks that have been tumble dried together and have become charged with static. The socks *can* be pulled apart, but the pulling will require a small amount of force: there is a perceptible magnetic attraction between the two socks.

A similar attraction may be palpable between your hands and the skin (even through clothing) of the partner. This feeling of magnetic attraction occurs when the patient or practice partner's skin or muscles *want* you to continue holding.

This feeling of magnetic attraction may occur before, during, and/or after the relaxation response.

Do not let go of your partner so long as you can feel that magnetic attraction that seems to be keeping your hands attached to your partner.

If you try to remove your hand while your hand is still being magnetically attracted to your partner's skin, it will feel as if you must use a bit of force, as if you are wrenching your hand up off of the partner. It will feel somehow wrong.

If you wait until the magnetic pull has dispersed, your hand will come up easily off of your partner. If the magnetic pull disperses and it feels as if the patient's skin has *reversed* its charge, your hand may almost feel as if it is being subtly repelled away from your partner.

If you feel as if your hand is being pushed away, then do not impose your hand any longer. Gently remove your hands. You are finished, at that location, at least for the time being.

Let go!

Sometimes, a Let go signal is *not* an indication that the relaxation response is finished. Sometimes, a person's skin will issue a "Let go" signal" immediately, even if there was *no* relaxation response. This behavior suggests that the partner is feeling very protective of this area. This may be an area that genuinely needs to be held, and will benefit from being held, but is not yet ready to be held. If this is the case, do not impose yourself on the area. Instead, the person might need to do some work to mentally turn off his dissociation and/or fear before you can work on the area.

You can move on. Your partner can work on turning off his dissociation or fear while you continue to assess his responsiveness elsewhere.

Choose another location a few inches away, and see if this new area is more willing to accept your hands' offer of support.

At some point, possibly after you've held the new spot for awhile, the partner's body may allow you to return to areas that previously didn't want you.

Of course, if the patient seems uneasy or begins verbally trying to distract you as you prepare to hold some part of his body, *don't* impose yourself. Try some other area first, and slowly win the confidence of the patient's subconscious at the same time that the patient is working on mentally changing his dissociation habit, if any.

Electric resistance to being touched

Sometimes, a person with strong emotional associations with his injury will have such strong resistance to being touched, particularly in the vicinity of an injured area, that when you first begin working with him, you *cannot* rest your hands on him for the first few minutes, or maybe the entire hour, of the treatment. It might feel as if a strong electrical charge is pushing you away. Sometimes this palpable resistance to being touched can be evident at every session for many weeks.

This extreme level of aversion to being touched in a supportive manner, even after doing mental exercises to terminate dissociation *might* mean that the person is using pause mode.

When I have a patient with this level of fear around being touched, I might do one of several things. I might place my hands on an area very far from the injured and resistant area. For example, if the injury is down in his foot, and his leg, all the way up to the hip, is pushing me away, I might hold his upper arm…if it will let me.

In a case like this, the best you might hope for in the first few sessions is letting the partner's body learn to trust your hands while you use them in a "safe" place: a place far away from the injury.

Or I might suspend my hands in the air space several inches immediately away from his injured body part. I support my hands with the muscles of my arms and shoulders, as if my hands were resting, nonchalantly, up against the electric field of his injured area that is emitting a powerful Let go! signal. Usually within a few minutes or a few weeks, the area is less afraid and allows me to set my hands down on the skin.

Then again, if this is the closest I can get to the partner, I might lead him through the steps for diagnosing pause (in the back of this book), at this point, to make sure that the patient is not using this neurological mode. If he is, I will *not* do FSR until pause has been turned off.

Taking too long to say "Let go"

Sometimes it will seem a bit awkward at first if you are working on a patient and a full minute goes by before you get the signal to let go. This awkwardness may be coming from completely unrelated social conventions that tell us not to shake someone's hand for too long, or not to hug a person for too long.

Please, if your skin feels as if it is adhering to the partner's body, don't worry about the social conventions for holding too long. If the patient's body wants continued contact, go ahead and give it.

The hug that lasts too long: an example

Oppositely, when you give a social hug that lasts too long, you can (if you are sensitive to these things) feel the electrostatic repulsion force coming from that person – even if you are both wearing heavy suits. Hopefully, most of us who are planning to do this type of work already know, via our intuition (which is to say, in this case, our awareness of the changes in static charge) exactly how long to keep hugging someone and when to let go.

Is there anyone among us who has not experienced an uncomfortable feeling after being hugged for a bit too long? Oppositely, haven't we all wanted, at some point in a harried or stressful day, to just be held tightly for an indefinite period – until we feel that we've had a chance to collect ourselves?

When holding small children, it is always obvious when they want to be held steadily and snugly. They snuggle in and almost burrow into your chest. And yet, the moment that they've decided that they don't need a hug anymore, they are impossible to restrain; they squirm and fidget, making it obvious that the time for holding is over. Period.

No one should need to be taught how to recognize when someone needs a hug, or when someone wants the hug to end. However, in our somewhat non-touching culture, when it comes to therapeutic touch, we actually have to study and practice in order to be able to perform these basic, human functions correctly.[1]

Working through clothing

Electromagnetic fields are not significantly inhibited by thin clothing, any more than the pull of a refrigerator magnet is significantly diminished by a thin piece of paper between the magnet and the door of the fridge.

The force of these fields *does* decrease over distance, whether or not there is clothing in the way. Therefore, thin clothing, which does not make a huge difference in the *distance* between your hands and the skin of your patient, will not diminish the signals being sent by the patient, but very *thick* clothing such as heavy parkas *can* diminish the sensations simply because it increases the *distance* between your hand and your partner's skin.

Relaxing all over

As you get more accustomed to paying attention to what is happening to the skin under your hands, you may notice a faint feeling of relaxation in your own hands, or even in your arms or torso, a feeling that occurs at the same instant that the magnetic clinging feeling goes away. As you become more comfortable doing this work, you may even begin to notice that your own body perceptibly relaxes at the same time as the partner's skin says "Let go."

Sometimes it can feel as if you had been unintentionally holding your breath, and at the moment when the partner relaxes, you find yourself exhaling, or relaxing your abdomen.

Review

When should you *not* let go? Do *not* let go as long as the feeling of being "stuck" to the partner's skin via magnetic attraction is ongoing. Do *not* let go if you feel as if your hands are being pulled in to the practice partner's skin. Do *not* let go if, when you try to remove your hands, you feel as if you have to use any force whatsoever to extricate your hands.

When *should* you let go? *Do* let go if the magnetism or subtle feeling of attraction has dispersed and you feel that you are no longer electrically attached to your partner's skin. *Do* let go if you feel an electric sense like that of two positive ends of a magnet being pushed at each other, repulsing each other, between your hands and your partner. *Do* let go if you feel uneasy in any way. Such a feeling of uneasiness may be coming from some

---

[1] Some people *do* have trouble recognizing these signals. I have noticed that people taking certain drugs, notably antidepressants, anti-anxiety drugs, and dopamine-enhancing anti-Parkinson's drugs, are sometimes not able to ascertain when they are receiving a Let go signal. And some people just seem to be insensitive to the signals from others, but it may be that this is learned behavior, and not a physiological lack.

Then again, genetic research in 2018 suggests that the capacity for empathy has a genetic component as well as being related to cultural influences. "Genone-wide analyses of self-reported empathy: correlations with autism, schoizophrenia, and anorexia nervosa"; Warrier, Toro, Bhakrabaris, et al, *Translational Psychiatry* DOI:10.1038/s41398-017-0082-6

energetic turmoil that has been stirred up in your patient, and, if you don't want to be a party to it, that's perfectly reasonable.

Of course, *do* let go if your partner verbally asks you to do so.

Working with a person with Parkinson's disease

When you first start practicing this type of therapy, you should *not* try to learn this awareness of when to let go by *first* working on a person with Parkinson's. The skin of a person with Parkinson's may repel you for months. Oppositely, it might not emit a Let Go signal for months. It may not do anything for a long, long time. The skin of a person with Parkinson's is the wrong place to learn sensitivity to shifts in electrical signals.

The absence of signals in the skin of a person with Parkinson's is closely related to the absence of signals in a mouse whose skin has been perforated by the claws of a cat: a mouse that has gone rigid and feels dead to the touch, a mouse that has slipped into the neurological mode of pause. The absence of electrical signal in the skin of the mouse contributes to the cat quickly developing a disinterest in the seemingly lifeless mouse.

I repeat, when you are first getting used to supportive holding and looking for signals regarding continuing the holding or letting go, practice on someone who does not have Parkinson's disease. You must first learn to recognize these feelings on a healthy person.

Then again, if you find that, right off the bat, your "Parkinson's" patient has normal, healthy responses to FSR treatment in his injured areas, there's a good chance your patient was misdiagnosed. He *might* not actually have idiopathic Parkinson's. Or maybe your Parkinson's patient has already read this material and turned off the dissociation or pause, and *that*'s why he's able to respond.

It is *possible* that your Parkinson's patient will give off attraction or repulsion signals but then again, it's *more* likely that he won't. At some point he may *begin* sending these electrical signals. That will be a good sign that things are going the right direction.

But, in the beginning, learn to recognize the basic human "Hold Me" magnetic attraction force or the Let go repulsion force while working on *healthy* people.

There are many cues that tell you whether to stay attached or to let go: the magnetic attraction (holding) force, the repellent (letting go) force, the partner's tension (which usually wants you to keep holding) or relaxation (often resulting in a Let go signal), and even a feeling of tension or relaxation somewhere deep within your own body. These are all signals telling you to either hang on or let go. You may notice one or several of them. When you feel *anything* telling you to let go, let go.

You are ready to Practice FSR

You now know the basic technique of FSR. It consists of:

1. Holding: first, ask permission. Then, hold supportively: in such a way that your hand's force is met with an opposing force by your opposite hand.

2. Follow: hold snugly enough to the person's skin with your hands so that if the skin or underlying tissues move, your hands move with them. You continue to give steady support.

3. Diagnose: If you get a response, even a flicker at the first moment, fine. Move on or, if there is a strong attraction between his skin and your hand, then wait for a Let go signal.

If the person's body does *not* respond to your holding, you might need to settle in for a long holding session at that location, or make a note of the location of the unresponsive area so that you can return to it later. This subject is discussed in greater detail in the next chapter.

4. Let go: when the patient's skin turns off or reverses the magnetic attraction to your hand, or when he verbally tells you to let go, then let go.

Get out there and practice

There is not very much about these techniques that can be taught in words. The techniques are very simple. The trick to mastering these techniques does not lie in intellectual understanding. The best way to become proficient is to jump right in and practice these biologically simple techniques. It is the practice, not the intellectual understanding, that will make you skilled.

So many students have told me, "I'm not sure what I'm feeling." The solution? Stop thinking about what you're feeling. *Thinking* about what the patient *might* need and *feeling* what the patient *does* need are two different things. Go with the feeling. Trust your hands.

Practice, practice, practice. At some point, you'll realize that your hands know what they are feeling, and they convey any pertinent information to your brain, without your analytical intelligence getting in the way.

Practice will teach you more than any words can.

Even a few hours of practice, on maybe half a dozen people, might be enough to teach you what a normal response is, and how to know when to let go. Even with this small amount of practice, you might soon be able to notice, through your hand's instincts, when something is "not right" and therefore wants to be held, firmly, calmly, with no intention on your part, until the area is ready to relax.

"Often the hands will solve a mystery that the mind has struggled with in vain."

– Carl Gustav Jung

Chapter ten

FSR as a diagnostic tool

Healthy areas in normal people usually relax quickly in response to firm, non-intentioned support. *Injured areas* in people who are guarded, dissociated, or on pause with regard to the injured area usually do *not* relax quickly in response to being firmly held.

This response, or lack of, allows you to use FSR as a diagnostic technique to determine where, exactly, an unhealed, dissociated or guarded injury, if any, is located. At the same time, FSR is a technique that can promote healing in such an area.

Referring to a health technique as both a diagnostic tool *and* a therapy is somewhat uncommon in the western medical realm. However, when applying assessment methods that indicate whether or not a person can pay attention to a given part of his body, the very process of assessment can also bring the patient's attention to that body part. As a person brings his attention or curiosity to an area, it may also bring healing capability to the area: so the health practitioner's assessment is also a contribution to the therapy.[1]

---

[1] Years ago, when I was studying Zero Balancing, a moderately Yin type of body stretching, the teacher kept saying "Gently move the patient's spine (or neck or whatever) in direction X or Y and then *assess* what happens." We were never told to treat anything – only "assess" the patient to see where work was needed. Over the course of two days, I got increasingly antsy with the "assessment" process. I was eager to find out what technique we would do on the areas that had been "assessed" as needing more work. It turns out, there *was no* treatment technique! The "assessment" was the whole thing.

Only at the end of the two-day workshop did it occur to me that the actual work of Zero Balancing *was* the gentle moving of the patient for "assessment" purposes: the assessment process was the technique. The verb "assess" had been used, very wisely, by the originator of Zero Balancing to prevent students from thinking that the imposed movements should *do* anything to the patient.

By asking practitioners to "assess" what happened when very gently stretching or moving the patient, the practitioners very carefully tuned in with what was going on in the patient's body, but didn't try to actively *do* any *intentional* "healing" therapy. The significant benefit that was observed by patients was "spontaneous": it occurred on its own, while the practitioners were very gently moving the patient around, making "assessments."

I came to understand, several years later, that a major challenge for the many founders of various schools of what's called "light touch" therapy is writing up the instructional material. If the founders use verbs that imply any sense of *doing* on the part of the practitioner, most of the students will cheerfully misunderstand and use some, and therefore, too much, willfull manipulation.

Diagnostically speaking, *if* your patient has a relaxation response to your firm support in some particular part of his body, then that body part is probably healthy enough, for your diagnostic purposes: you probably don't need to work any longer in that particular area.

Even so, hold it until it tells you to let go. It will probably tell you to let go very quickly, in a few seconds or so.

If there *had been* any lurking unhealed bits of displaced bone or twisted fascia in the area, the relaxation response and the anti-magnetic (the repulsion) "Let go" response will indicate that your partner's brain is 1) aware of your presence and 2) may have been successfully reminded to start healing any unfinished business. The body might still have some healing to do, but *your* job is finished: you have brought the patient's awareness to the area.

If your patient or practice partner did have a quick relaxation response, you can make a mental note of the fact that this particular body location is *able* to respond, and you can move on to the next body location, which might be a few inches away or somewhere else entirely.

For diagnostic purposes, we are not necessarily looking for any specific sort of movement. What we are looking for is the ability to respond in some manner – *any* manner. If an area is mentally blocked or dissociated, it will *not* be able to respond to your touch. If it cannot respond, it also cannot fully heal. If it cannot respond, you want to know about it, so that you can plan on spending time holding that body part. You might do the FSR holding now, or you might just make a note of the rigidity and come back later, after doing more assessment.

Watching for movement

Practice supportive holding on your partner's forearm and notice whether or not any response occurs, and if so, how much. This may seem redundant at this point, but though this action is similar to what you did in a previous chapter, notice that the focus has now changed. We have moved away from "How much pressure?" to "Was there a relaxation response?"

As pointed out in chapter eight and shown in the photographs labeled Fig.8.1 and 8.2, the relaxation response can be very very quick, and very subtle. You set your hands on your patient in a specific position and almost instantly, in most cases, your hands are in a slightly different position because the patient's muscles have moved into a more relaxed position.

So even though you have already practiced holding, try it again, but this time stay focused on whether or not your patient responds. If he does respond, make a mental note that this area is OK, and move on to another spot.

You can ask your practice partner if he has a history of broken arm or other trauma in the arm. If so, this will be a good place to practice holding. There is a good chance that the injured area will *not* respond as quickly, if at all, as other parts of the arm – a learning experience.

If you still have gotten no relaxation response after a few minutes nor a Let go signal (as discussed in the previous chapter), if the area just feels sort of dead, like the proverbial "bump on a log," lift your hands off the skin and move them to a new location a few inches away. See if this new location responds.

If, at the new place, you get no response or you get another Let go signal, move to yet another location. Very often, when working on a foot injury, the nearest place that will actually respond is much farther up the leg, maybe even the at the thigh.

When you finally get to a place on the patient's body that has a relaxation response to your holding, you now have a starting place from you can slowly advance into the unresponsive area. You hold the responsive area until it tells you to let go. You let go and move an inch or so into the previously unresponsive area. You stay there until you get a "let go" response.

Repeat this slow, steady progress into the next unresponsive area. Continue until the entire area is able to respond to your supportive holding. When you are holding directly over the most injured area you might need to hold for half an hour or even more. How long the patient remains unresponsive depends a lot on the degree to which the patient has been working on making himself mentally available to the area: the degree to which the patient has turned off any dissociation or the use of pause.

By practicing FSR on a healthy person, you can learn to quickly recognize what the normal range of responses of a healthy person feel like. Then, when you work on a person who has an injury, you will be able to recognize the pathological response of rigidity, lack of relaxation or an immediate Let go signal. Sometimes, you might not even be able to put your hands on the patient in the area you are aiming for, because the patient's skin in that area is giving off a signal of magnetic repulsion before you even physically touch the area.

The lightening fast response

As noted previously, students often assume the response will not occur for several seconds. They ignore that first, instantaneous "flinching" movement, and settle in to watch for something dramatic.

The tiny "flinch" may well be the reflexive relaxation response that you are looking for.

Working with a person with Parkinson's

When treating a person with Parkinson's disease, in order to discover which areas of his legs and feet do *not* respond with a somewhat normal reflexive movement, FSR is first used on his legs and feet in a fairly quick manner, looking for an area that will do *any* sort of response. Very often, even if the foot and ankle are not responsive, a relaxation response *can* be felt up by the knee, or in more "stuck" cases, up above the knee, on the thigh or even the hip. After finding some spot on the hip, thigh, knee, or lower leg that *is* responsive, you can then move down the leg, a few inches at a time, until you get to a spot that *doesn't* respond to your holding. You can then stay at this location until it responds, until it "releases" the tension.

You can work your way from an area that *is* responsive down into an area of the patient's foot or leg (and later on, possibly an arm, hip, shoulder, neck, or cranial bone) that does *not* respond within a few moments, or minutes. At this point, you might decide that you are done with diagnosing, for now. Instead, you can settle in to provide "treatment" in some particular location, usually an unresponsive area that is immediately adjacent to a responsive area. You can settle in, get comfortable, and just hold the area until it responds.

The response, the release of its rigid holding pattern, might come in minutes, or in hours, or after a few months of once-a-week, one-hour treatments. If the practitioner is a spouse or a friend that lives nearby, treatments might be given every day. Usually, you don't want to do this for more than one hour per day.

Broken bones

Several times, when I've worked on a *severely* immobile area and it has finally relaxed, the patient has later on, within minutes or days, experienced the severe pain of the original injury. Often, within a few days, bruising and swelling suggestive of a broken bone(s) appears. Sometimes, the patient has then recalled an event from decades earlier that probably caused the break.

In some cases, after a week or so of extreme pain, patients have then gotten radiology work done. Their scans have revealed broken bones.

Sometimes, because the bone break shows a week's worth of healing, the patient is admonished by the radiologist, "You should have come in a week ago, when you broke this. I can see there is a week's worth of healing at the edges of the break."

If the patient tries to explain that the bone was broken *years* ago but only started doing healing a week ago, the radiologist might assume the patient is lying. (This is what my patients report to me.) Regardless, once the healing has started, it will proceed to fully heal.

Having radiology work isn't necessary, of course. But this secondary form of diagnostics, radiology, can be helpful in proving to the patient that he *did*, in fact, have a significant unhealed injury. This knowledge can help a patient be more patient with the healing process.[1]

Setting standards for diagnostic tools: determining what is normal

You *must* practice on healthy people before undertaking treatment of people with Parkinson's or other syndromes that are related to dissociation or trauma. You must become familiar with what constitutes a "healthy" response. A short vignette will demonstrate the importance of this.

---

[1] When I had barely started doing Yin Tui Na, my daughter broke a bone in her foot. The after-hours doctor to which I took her was *not* a radiologist. He took an x-ray, glanced at it, and told me the foot bone *wasn't* broken.

I replied that I knew that it was broken based on Asian medicine diagnostics. In this case, I was basing my diagnosis on both FSR *and* the sudden sensitivity in my daughter's acupoint UB-11, a point near the spine at the level of the first rib, a point known as "the meeting point for the bones."

The doctor was unsettled enough by my confident attitude that, next morning, he showed the x-ray to an actual radiologist. The radiologist quickly pointed to the break, at the exact location that I had described. The doctor, who had a Chinese surname, was kind enough to call me and tell me that I'd been right, and went on to say that he had always been fascinated by Asian medicine.

*"My patients don't feel like *this*!"*

My first weekend FSR seminar was attended by health practitioners, mostly licensed acupuncturists, who had already started using FSR on their patients with Parkinson's disease (PD).

These practitioners were self-taught in FSR. They had used an earlier edition of this text as their training manual. And for the most part, *despite* my admonitions, they had *never* worked on healthy people – people with normal responses.

Most of them felt that they'd already treated their PD patients "long enough" (a mere few weeks or maybe a couple of months) and wondered why they weren't seeing some recovery symptoms.

I repeat, most of these practitioners had never bothered to practice first on healthy people. Ignoring the text's repeated suggestions that these techniques should be first practiced on healthy people, these practitioners had assured themselves that the tiny, random, once-in-a-great while sensations of faint electrical static coming from their Parkinson's patients were the normal relaxation responses that they were looking for.

Based on this wrong, presumed "evidence" of relaxation responses, they all had assumed that their patients' injuries must have started healing.

The therapists, being acupuncturists, for the most part, had moved on from using FSR based on these faint sensations of static coming from terribly rigid and unresponsive feet and ankles, and were now using acupuncture needles (their comfort zone) or physical manipulations on people who still had unhealed, dissociated injuries or were on pause *and* who still had the backwards-running channel Qi that is characteristic of Parkinson's.

I quickly learned that these acupuncturists were all using needles to try to invigorate the currents of channel Qi, despite their patients' currents still running backwards. They assumed that this was the right course because the blockage *must* be gone: it must be gone because they had spent *hours* doing FSR and they had felt *faint* sensations of static, which they assumed was the same as *relaxation movements*: releases of holding patterns.

(This was prior to 2003, when we were still working with people that were taking anti-parkinson's medications. The static feeling, and/or a feeling as if snakes are moving under the skin is characteristic in people using dopamine-enhancing medications.)

They thought that, with effort, they could detect subtle static, or maybe movement deep inside the skin. Because there were no other responses occurring, they assumed, wrongly, that these bits of static charge must be the "relaxation movement" that I'd written about.

During the seminar, I had the students begin by working on each other – working on relatively healthy people.

When the students settled their hands on healthy people, their fellow students, they were astonished.

One student exclaimed to the room at large, "Oh my gosh! Is this what a normal person responds like? This is a *huge* response! My Parkinson's patient doesn't feel *anything* like this!"

This particular practitioner had been writing to me for about two months telling me about her FSR progress with her PD patient. She had said that he was responding beautifully to her FSR, but he wasn't seeing a change in his PD symptoms. She wondered why.

When this practitioner exclaimed this way, I asked her point blank if she had *ever* tried these techniques on a healthy person – as repeatedly recommended in my previous editions of this material.

She told me, "No, I assumed I didn't need to. I'm a licensed acupuncturist, and a massage therapist. I thought I knew what it felt like to touch a person."

As a massage therapist, she *did* know what it felt like, to her, to invasively push and shove on a person. But she'd *never* paid much attention to how the patient *responded*. She had *never* noticed how a patient *responds* to supportive, non-invasive holding.

In fact, with all the students at the seminar, their Parkinson's patients were *not* yet making normal responses to touch, but the students assumed that they *were*. Their patients still needed lots of Yin Tui Na therapy. For that matter, many were actually stuck on pause or dissociated. They needed *more* than just FSR. They needed to do mental work to either re-associate with the injury or turn off their use of pause mode.

But the main point here is that the therapists, even those with years of experience in bodywork of the push-and-shove variety didn't have any idea what a healthy and normal *relaxation* response was.

Oppositely, when I taught a class at the local acupuncture college, a class in general Yin Tui Na, using FSR as the *most* Yin example of Tui Na techniques, my students quickly, within a few weeks of practicing FSR on each other, felt *very* confident that they knew how to supportively hold a patient and observe the quick relaxation response.

After a few weeks, I brought into class, as subjects, six people with Parkinson's, so that my students could learn how to do the very patient, slow part of this technique: sitting and holding and waiting for a response from a person whose body *doesn't* want to respond with relaxation, at first.

Within a few minutes of snuggling their hands onto the legs and/or feet of the people with Parkinson's, all the students looked baffled.

One raised her hand, "What is it we're supposed to be doing?"

The other students quickly chimed in. "I've forgotten what we're supposed to do!" and "I've forgotten what we're looking for!"

The utter non-responses, the deathlike stillness in feet of people with Parkinson's were *so* weird, so *completely* abnormal, that all of the students felt that they'd "forgotten" what it was they were supposed to be doing.

I had to reassure the students that they were doing the technique correctly – the non-response was because of the patients, *not* because of the poor technique of the students.

Even though the patients were not responding to being held, the job of the students was to find some area farther up the leg that might be *capable* of a healthy response.

Then, they needed to provide supportive holding until such time as the patient's rigidity relaxed or gave a Let go signal, or until the patient starting being a little responsive in any way, shape, or form. Then, after that response, they might move their hands a little further into the non-responsive zone.

If a person has no training in FSR, he may not realize if a patient is having a somewhat "normal" response or not. Therefore, I state again: the following techniques should be practiced on several healthy people before they are used on people with injury-induced rigidity, pain, numbness, or some sort of "holding pattern."

After practicing these techniques on several or dozens of healthy people, a therapist may have enough sense of the normal range of healthy response that, when he comes across a strangely unresponsive area on his patient, he will be able to suspect that there is something wrong, such as unhealed injury, or even dissociation, at that spot. He will also be able to tell when the injured area is starting to feel healthier, closer to normal, because it will eventually begin to relax, to move, in response to support.

"Never tonify a rebellious condition"

As an aside to any acupuncturist reading this book and a follow up to the above section that mentioned acupuncturists using needles on patients who weren't "ready," you might recall from your schooling that inserting acupuncture needles into backwards flowing channel Qi will *not* correct the flow pattern. It is a first-semester rule of Chinese medicine that one should "Never Tonify an Excess condition."

"Stagnation," channel Qi (electrical) blockages, and the backwards-running ("Rebellious") channel Qi that is characteristic of Parkinson's are all "Excess" conditions.

Inserting acupuncture needles into an area that is Excess increases the amperage (Tonifies) in the immediate vicinity of the needles, and can *increase* the amount of current that is Stagnant, blocked, or running backwards, thus making things worse.

Don't *ever* insert needles in a current that is running backwards.[1]

Immobility and non-responsiveness coming from the mind, with no injury

In some cases, FSR will elicit no response, whatsoever – as *if* the patient has an unhealed injury from which he has dissociated – but there is no injury anywhere in the body, none at all. The patient just has a profound inability to respond.

This kind of non-responsiveness is, in my experience, most often an indication that the person is using pause mode. The use of pause can trigger the non-responsiveness that is *supposed* to occur when a person is in profound shock or coma, teetering on the verge of death.

Essential tremor

I have seen patients with no history of any significant injury, whose bodies do not feel as if they are suppressing an injury, who are using self-induced pause. These patients have often had terrible tremoring, especially in the hands and arms, but they do not have the four categories of symptoms necessary to make a diagnosis of Parkinson's. They have usually been diagnosed with Essential Tremor.

Unlike most of my patients with Parkinson's, whose diagnostic visualizations suggest agitation in the area of the sacrum, some people with essential tremor have diagnostic visualizations that suggest agitation in the pericardium, the connective tissue around the heart.

---

[1] *Tracking the Dragon*, a textbook on advanced channel theory, goes into this in great detail. Available at JaniceHadlock.com. The first chapter is available for free download at www.pdrecovery.org.

Some weirdnesses of partial recovery

Sometimes, if the person is in partial recovery, he may perform "normal" relaxation responses if his mindset switches over to "relaxed" (not on pause).

I can often induce such a fleeting "mental relaxation" in a person with partial recovery from Parkinson's by telling a goofy joke or two. I tell the joke, and within less than a minute, the leg or foot becomes responsive. As soon as the patient has time to revert back to his usual mindset of pause, complete with a high level of risk-assessment and wariness, the leg may become unresponsive again – either immediately or over the next hour or so.

A patient who is using self-induced pause to "keep himself safe" may learn to relax during FSR sessions: the leg or foot in question will relax and be responsive during treatments, but it can tighten back up and *behave as if injured* again as soon as the treatment session is over. I had one patient whose legs stay relaxed for a day and a half, following each FSR session, before tightening back up again from fear. This patient did not need more FSR, though he liked getting it. He needed to turn off his self-induced pause – which he did *not* want to do.

He wanted *me* to permanently turn off his mental use of pause by holding his *feet* once a week. This is impossible. The root of the problem was in his own mind, not in his foot.

In response to each week's FSR session, he was able to move normally for hours or even a day or two, until some negative thought passed through his mind, after which he had all his symptoms of Parkinson's again.

Again, if your patient is stuck in partial recovery or is still using self-induced pause, your use of FSR for the legs and feet might be met with rigidity and non-responsiveness even though there is *no injury-based blockage*. In some cases, there *was* an injury, the injury responded to FSR, and the injury has now healed *but* the patient will *still* revert into rigidity – *exactly* as if re-injured – in the *healed* area…because he is still using self-induced pause. This is another example of the bizarre things that can happen in partial recovery.

The solution in this case is *not* more FSR. The only solution is turning off pause – and it will be harder to turn off pause if the injury has been treated with FSR and then healed while the mind was still using the wariness of pause: was still obeying an instruction to pretend to be numb or as if on the verge of death.

As noted in chapter three, a person who is stuck on pause is *not* a good candidate for FSR treatment until after he turns off the pause behaviors and his body behaves physiologically and electrically as if he feels inherently safe enough to be fully alive. He may be worse off if his injury(s) heal while he is still on pause.

Multiple injuries

You might find more than one place on the body that needs attention.

In one memorable case, a professional musician who had Parkinson's from dissociation, a person who was *not* on pause, was still manifesting many Parkinson's symptoms even after she re-associated with her foot injury. After her foot injury healed, her *legs* resumed normal, healthy movement. However, she still had tremor and rigidity in her face and arms.

Like many of my other Parkinson's patients who were professional musicians, she had dissociated from her injuries but had *not* put herself on pause.

Despite her legs resuming normal function, she still seemed to have what you might call constant, "full-blown Parkinson's" in her upper body. This was very unlike those patients who are on pause who slide into partial recovery after the foot injury has healed.

A thorough inquiry revealed that, about ten years earlier, she had received a violent blow to the side of the head from a piece of falling furniture: she'd been unconscious for two days.

I was baffled because her Parkinson's symptoms weren't completely clearing up now that her foot injury had healed. So I decided to hold the site of the old head injury. I had been firmly holding her utterly rigid temporal bones (near the ears). These bones, derived from ancestral gills, are supposed to perform a faint back and forth rotation with every incoming and outgoing breath. I'd been holding these unmoving bones, simply holding them with firm, supportive pressure, for around forty-five minutes when, suddenly, it felt to my hands as if all the bones in her skull were shifting around.

Right there in my office, she experienced the recovery symptom of internal brain shift that's described in *Recovery from Parkinson's*. All her symptoms utterly ceased. The *internal* tremor, as well as the visible tremor, disappeared. Her neck relaxed, straightened out, and then, though her face had been a rigid mask a few minutes earlier, she smiled!

And she announced, with utter certainty, "I'm all better!"

And she was.

That was more than ten years ago, and she's not had any Parkinson's symptoms since that day.

I included this case study to make the point that sometimes, as you are looking for an area that is unresponsive and possibly dissociated, there might be *more* than one place that wants holding.

Diagnostics based on some sort of response: summary

This technique can be used diagnostically in this sense: if no response occurs in the patient within a few seconds of making contact, there is probably subconscious tension, physical or electrical blockage, or some sort of mental protective holding pattern such as dissociation or self-induced dissociation in the vicinity of where you are holding, *or* the use of pause mode.

Again, what is a relaxation response? Any movement. The movement may be almost visually imperceptible, or it might be a big jerk. It may be accompanied by a small clicking or popping sound as bones slide back into place. Movements might seem like the follow-through to an old impact, or wiggle back and forth, or make circular movements, or a slow glide. The response might occur almost instantly, and you might even miss it unless you are paying attention, or it might take a few seconds, or even up to a minute.

Oppositely, an *absence* of movement *or* a subtle magnetic attraction between your hand and the patient's skin, an attraction that doesn't want to let go even after ten minutes, or longer, suggests that there's something either out of place, broken, or for some other reason crying for attention in the immediate area. But it's not yet ready or able to respond and/or release. If so, this area may benefit from a short or a long period of holding, or several sessions of holding – sessions that eventually lead up to one, or several, relaxation responses.

If you use this technique regularly, you may become very accurate in your diagnoses: quickly able to determine the exact locations of unhealed injuries – including ones of which the patient is not aware (although he or family members might remember it when asked.) For that matter, I've had patients who were unaware of ever having a foot injury even though they had a large surgical scar, complete with the little dots where the sutures were, on their foot. Only after they re-associated with their feet were they able to say something like, "Hey, look! There's a scar there. I just remembered when that happened…"

And if you use this technique often enough, you will prove to yourself that you *can* help initiate healing in a rigid or unhealed area by giving a person's injury(s) the supportive holding that it has been waiting for.

Chapter eleven

Advanced FSR techniques

Holding combined with a bit of a nudge

Sometimes, if the person's body does not respond immediately to firm, supportive contact, it is possible that, instead of stony dissociation, only some mild tension is stubbornly residing therein. Very often, in these cases, the area under contact will not budge until some gentle suggestion of movement disrupts the tension pattern. The area, even if it doesn't move *instantly*, *might* move and respond if it is given a little bit of a nudge.

Sometimes, a slight nudge of movement from the practitioner's hands is all that is required for the body part in question to wake up to the fact that it is being supported. Once it is awake, the body part may respond nicely.

As soon as you make a tiny move, the patient's subconscious muscle tension might loosen up enough that, a moment or two later, it *will* respond to your continuation of the simple firm holding of FSR by making some relaxation movement.

Even without the presence of dissociation or an unhealed injury, a patient may have some little bit of hesitancy or tension, some snag in a certain area that prevents relaxation of that area. If a patient's body does not seem to respond in any way to being supported, a gentle, almost imperceptible nudge, even an *imagined* nudge of your hands may be enough to suggest to the patient's muscle tension that he can let go of the snag. If so, you will perceive a slight relaxation movement in response to the nudge.

Then, after the initial hesitancy is gone, the patient may respond further or, in future, he will respond normally to the basic holding technique.

Diagnostically, if this spot is able to respond to a small nudge of the hands, this spot was *not* what you would call a "problem area." Diagnostically, the area *was* able to respond. As a diagnostician, you are mostly hunting for areas that do not respond to holding *or* to a gentle nudge. As soon as an area responds, the practitioner can either move along or wait for a Let go signal.

A bit of a nudge

What is meant by a bit of a nudge or a *tiny* nudge?

The tiny movement is not really a push, it is more like a tiny bounce, or pulsing motion in which the practitioner's hands move, momentarily, a sixteenth (1/16) or a thirty-second (1/32) of an inch closer together and then rebound back apart again.

Let's say that you, the practitioner, find yourself supporting your partner's forearm with your hands opposite each other. You may employ a little bit of quick force to bring your hands closer together ever-so-slightly. Then, *immediately* let your hands rebound back to their original position.

Note that I never use the words "push or shove on the *patient* with your hands." Instead, my language is that the hands of the practitioner come closer to each other and then bounce back apart to their starting position. The practitioner is focusing on his own hands, *not* on what is happening to the patient.

If this tiny bit of a nudge is small enough, the patient will not even perceive the force of the nudge. The nudge will not be felt because both of your hands are opposite each other, taking up the nudge pressure from each other. Since the patient is supported, he doesn't need to do any work to resist the change in pressure. Therefore, he won't really notice what you are doing.

Very often, if a slight tension in the patient is preventing the normal type of relaxation response that most people have to supportive holding, this tiny, very quick, invisible-to-the-naked-eye nudging movement, or maybe five or six nudging movements, will dislodge the tension. Once the tension is dislodged, the area being held may well move a bit in one direction or another. Then, the area may take advantage of the support being provided to relax to a yet more comfortable position. When this occurs, when the area starts to move, the practitioner's hands must follow the movement, continuing to provide support, as described in the section on holding on, until the hands get a Let go signal.

If nothing happens: *imagine* the nudge

Sometime, when the area is stubborn and doesn't even flinch or move in response to a subtle, quick nudge, you need to become *more* subtle. In such cases, *imagining* that you are pulsing your hands together for a fleeting moment might elicit a response.

Bear in mind that you are *not* imagining that the *patient* is going to move. This would be an imposition on the patient. As always, this technique allows the patient to do whatever he wants. You will imagine only that *your* hands are moving closer together, just a tad, and then rebounding to their original position.

This extremely subtle type of "movement" (imaginary) is very often the most effective type of stimulation for stubborn tensions. Very often, *imagining* that you are moving your hands as if giving a tiny nudge is the best way to wake up an area in your partner that is stubbornly stuck.

If nothing happens: change hand positions

If there is no response to the little pulsing movement of your hands, or several of them, you can either just stay where you are and, giving firm support, try another nudge in a few minutes, or you can move the hands a little bit, to a new position. Maybe move them a little more anteriorly/posteriorly (fore and aft), or maybe a little bit laterally/medially (side to side).

Play around with responding to what you feel in your patient. This is not a precise rocket science. What you are doing with FSR is merely giving support to a person in a very natural way, in the same way a dog will automatically know to lick his owner at the owner's injury site.

The only reason this subject has to be addressed in a book is that we have been taught to *not* touch ourselves or others in a healing way, and we've been taught to *ignore* our intuitive awareness of how another person is best able to accept physical support.

You can learn to do this. Mostly, you just need to *unlearn* your hesitancy and listen to your own hands.

If nothing happens: try something else

You can try a few other moves with your hands if there is no response even after you try doing a gentle, two-handed nudge or an imaginary nudge. You can try shifting your hands a bit: maybe they will settle into a position that is even more comfortable for *you*, and which therefore conveys a more supportive feeling to your *partner*.

If nothing you do elicits a response, you can try again, using a slightly more *forceful* nudge. Every once in a very great while, a genuine physical move of pushing your hands together a whopping fourth of an inch (1/4") with an actual bit of force and then immediately letting your hands rebound to the original position *might* be beneficial and might trigger a response and relaxation from the person's rigid body part.

Usually, if this is the case, you will know it because something in your hands "tells you" that a slight amount of physical "bouncing" or "nudging" is necessary.

In general, using more force is a technique of last resort, but once in a while, you might feel the need to do so. If so, don't be overtly pushy, of course. Simply bring your hands together a tiny bit more crisply than usual, using a tiny bit more force, and let them bounce back again to their normal holding position.

If this extra force doesn't do any good, it's usually best to go back to simple holding for a few more minutes to see if any sort of response will occur. If, after a bit of pulsing movements with your hands, either small or slightly forceful, nothing happens, then you can conclude that you've found a "stuck place." Settle in and just hold the area.

Or, very possibly, after the *surrounding* areas have relaxed, the stubborn area will be able to respond.

If the stubborn bit simply does not respond no matter what, but instead sits impassively, as if it isn't really quite alive, it is very likely that an injury, subconscious tension and/or tissue displacement has happened in this area, together with dissociation or the use of pause mode. If this is the case, and you are still just doing diagnostic assessment, you will want to make a written or mental note of the area, and then move on.

If you have already assessed the whole area and you are returning to those areas that didn't seem to respond, then make yourself comfortable and settle down to holding this unresponsive area for a long, long time, while maybe walking your patient through the exercises for turning off dissociation or self-induced dissociation.

Again, help in diagnosing which type of mental situation is present, if any, is provided at the back of this book in the appendices.

Advanced techniques for Parkinson's patients

When working on a Parkinson's patient, it is *very* likely that you will find unresponsive areas in the ankle and mid-foot. You might also find unresponsive areas in the knee, hip, shoulder, neck, and other areas, depending on the injury history of your patient.

Working with a person with Parkinson's can be a bit more challenging than working with a non-PD patient, because the areas that are unresponsive can cover such a large part of the body.

For example, if the PD patient dissociated from his foot when he was a child, the non-responsive area may have slowly and surreptitiously expanded to include his ankle, lower leg, knee, and even upper leg or hip. By the time you start working on the patient, his entire leg may feel somewhat dead, wooden, and unresponsive. But you don't really want to be holding the upper leg for an hour a week, for a year, when the actual unhealed injury location is in the foot.

So you will want to feel over the entire unresponsive area to find that spot that feels the *most* rigid.

I usually start up by the knee – assuming that there are signs of responsiveness in the knee area. After holding the knee for a bit, until it responds, I'll place my hands a few inches below the knee, and wait for a response. If there is a response, I'll move my hands even lower down the leg, and keep going until I get to a rigid place.

If, on the other hand, the place just below the knee shows no signs of response, I may choose to stay there for five or ten minutes, just to see what happens, and to give the body a chance to get used to the idea of being held in my hands. Sometimes, after ten minutes or so, the leg area being held will respond in some manner and I will continue working my way down the leg. Other times, it will not respond at all.

If this is the case, I will give a gentle nudge, a gentler nudge, an imaginary nudge, and maybe a slightly stronger nudge. If there has been no response, I might *still* continue a few inches down the leg again, slowly making my way towards the spot that is more *probably* the source of the original problem: the ankle and/or foot.

With people with Parkinson's, I often find that *imagining* a nudging movement in my hands is just as likely, or even more likely, to elicit a response than *actual* movement of my hands. Then again, every patient is different.

When I finally arrive at what is most likely the real source of the problem – the actual location of injury, the original point of impact – the area usually feels truly different. It just feels *wrong*. You can only know what feels wrong, of course, if you have spent some time learning what feels *right*.

One way in which the location might feel wrong is that bones are obviously displaced – sticking out from the usual line of the foot, or the whole foot may be jutting to one side or the other, due to a displacement in the ankle. These visually obvious displacements can be helpful. But after you've done this work for a while, the non-visible, *feel*-able vibrations given off by a displaced or damaged body part are your best diagnostic cues.

Once I get to the place where the actual injury is probably lurking, I settle in and get comfortable. Often, my approach is to start with just holding at the injury site. This is most often, because of the design of the foot, located at the second cuneiform bone, in the center of the foot. I hold that area for maybe ten minutes, maybe fifty minutes.

If there has been no response after about ten minutes, I might make very small moves with my hands. If there is no response, my hand movements get smaller still. Always, my goal is to be firm yet fairly imperceptible to the patient.

If still no response, I might make an even tinier movement. If still no response, I will try to keep my hands stationary and *imagine* that I am making a tiny movement. If this doesn't work, I will imagine that I am making an even tinier movement. If, after all this, there has been no response, I go back to just plain holding, firmly, for another ten minutes or half hour or fifty minutes – whatever seems right at the time. I never do more than a one-hour session. I usually work with a patient once a week, for an hour at a time.

Sometimes, a patient's body can produce a Let go signal even though nothing "positive" has happened. When this occurs, let go, and hold on somewhere else, nearby. This is not a bad thing – it shows that the patient *did* have some awareness of your hands, even if it was only a resentful one. That might signify progress.

Other times, it may seem as if the patient's injured foot or ankle is pulling your hands deeper into his skin, as if he desperately wants even more support than you are giving. This, too, is a response, and therefore a good thing. If you get this powerful feeling that your hands are being "sucked in" to the patient's skin, then stay where you are and let your hands stick like glue until the feeling shifts or the session comes to a close.

Then again, if the patient's *foot* has the injury but the upper *leg* or *knee* is pulling you in, for support, don't necessarily spend all your time on that upper leg or knee. Be sure to spend more of your time on the root of the problem – usually the ankle and/or foot.

When the foot finally does start to respond and the bones or tendons reposition themselves or release static charge into your hands, the upper leg might very well automatically get the energy and flexibility that it's been yearning for.

With PD patients, you probably want to spend most of your time on the foot and/or ankle, even though other areas are calling to you. In the end, it is *usually*, though not always, the foot/ankle problem that is causing the upper leg and knee problems.

This is not always the case. I had one patient whose foot and ankle problems were pretty much resolved, after about two years of once-a-week, one-hour treatments. However, she still had rigidity in her leg and hip, so I started focusing on these areas. After a year of holding her unresponsive leg, one hour sessions, one per week, her thigh began to move in response to my holding. *Excruciating* pain erupted in her upper leg. Within a day, a massive, blackish bruise appeared. It covered half of the side of her thigh, the type of bruise you might expect from a broken femur (thigh bone). The pain and the bruise slowly dissipated over several weeks. She could not bear weight on that leg during this time. Slowly, the area healed.

She probably needed FSR therapy over such a long span because I had not yet learned about mental medical Qi Gong exercises to accelerate getting rid of dissociation and pause, both of which she had, as it turned out. I had been using only Yin Tui Na.

But the main point here is that, *if* there is an injury in the knee or leg, in addition to the foot injury, those injuries might also need hands-on support.

But many, maybe most, people with PD have only the foot and/or ankle injury holding the PD symptoms in place – together with dissociation and/or in most cases, pause.

You just never know exactly what might be hidden inside the body of a person who has led an active life and who, since childhood has been dissociating from injuries or telling himself to "play dead" or "don't feel."

Getting back to the amount of nudging that you might do: if there has been no response to any of the nudgings, don't try them again right away. It may require weeks, even months, of holding treatments before the injury in a person with Parkinson's becomes responsive. Too much nudging and messing around can actually cause increased guardedness in the person with Parkinson's, and increase the total amount of time needed for therapy.

Don't stare down your patient's unblinking foot

Don't forget: your attention is on your own hands and not particularly focused on the patient. Don't be scrutinizing the patient too severely. Don't be impatient. It's not up to you when a person is going to decide that he's safe enough to deal with his past injuries.

A watched pot never boils and a wary person, like a silverback gorilla, does not like to be stared at. You can learn to be aware of whether or not a patient has responded without conveying to the patient that his every move is being assessed.

Be somewhat detached, but firm in your connection, like the sailor that shifts and sways ever so slightly in response to the movement of the ocean, even though he is not paying conscious attention to the waves.

Chapter twelve

Foot and ankle work

This chapter has some specific holding suggestions for ankle and foot.

The drawings of the foot bones in this chapter might help you feel more familiar with the terrain as you start to hold your patients feet. The first drawing is a top view of the foot, with each of the bones labeled. This drawing, a simplified diagram of the foot bones, is provided to familiarize you with the names of the bones and their approximate locations.

The detailed, dimensional drawings of the foot bones are viewed from seven different angles. The detailed diagrams give a better sense of how the joints actually fit together in three dimensions.

Regarding people with Parkinson's

Although people with Parkinson's may have neck, shoulder, hip, arm, cranial and spinal injuries that will benefit from treatment, and all of them *might* need to be treated in order to recover, they almost *always* have foot injuries. Not only that, if the foot injury is causing a blockage at the intermediate cuneiform bone or vicinity, it is contributing to, or in some cases of dissociation, solely responsible for, those backwards-flowing electrical currents that are seen in idiopathic Parkinson's.

Sometimes other foot and ankle injuries also contribute. Still, based on what seems to be the most frequent site for injured and displaced tissues, after exploring the general area and finding the areas that are unresponsive, I usually end up starting my long-term holding with the almost-always-present Unhealed Foot Injury at the intermediate cuneiform.

Even if the foot starts to heal on its own as soon as pause or dissociation has been turned off, I still like to start treating a Parkinson's patient at the 2nd cuneiform bone, one of the foot bones with the widest range of movement, and therefore the one most likely to be displaced in a foot injury.

Notice the intermediate cuneiform bone

As you peruse the drawings, particularly note the size and shape of the middle (the 2nd, or "intermediate") cuneiform bone in all the drawings. This center-of-the foot bone is supposed to move up and down freely during every footfall, enabling the foot to be somewhat arched or flat, at any given moment. Because of its tremendous freedom of movement, this bone is the one that is most often displaced during foot injuries.

This bone marks the end of an electrical sub-dermal current referred to, in Chinese medicine, as the "Stomach channel." This bone is the point from which the Stomach channel bifurcates, one branch flowing down to the toes, another branch flowing over to the side of the foot. Obstructions to electrical flow in the vicinity of this bone, obstructions such as torn or displaced tissue, scar tissue, and emotional inhibitions, can cause the Stomach channel to reverse course and run *backwards* – run *up* the leg.

Also, during healthy, normal use of pause mode due to severe shock, coma, or life-threatening injury, it is from this point on the foot that the energy in the Stomach channel flows backwards, moving towards the head.[1]

Observe that this intermediate cuneiform bone is quite substantial when looking down on it from the top view of the foot (fig. 12.1 and fig. 12.4). It looks like a good-sized "square" bone. The view of the same bone from the underside (plantar side) of the foot (fig. 12.8) will show you that this bone is so severely wedge-shaped from top to bottom that it tapers nearly to the point of disappearance by the time it gets to the underside of the foot; all that can be seen of it is a tiny sliver, tucked almost under the 1st cuneiform bone.

The word "cuneiform" means "wedge-shaped.

"Ankle bones"

In the drawings that follow, the so-called "ankle bones" are not pictured. To be perfectly accurate, the so-called "ankle bones" are protrusions on the lower *leg* bones. These knobby ends of the leg bones nestle into either side of the talus bone, as well as sticking out to the sides, forming the protrusions that we refer to as "ankle bones."

---

[1] As a physiological aside, the backwards flow of the Stomach channel Qi during pause mode is the reason that nausea is a common side-effect of shock or body-wide anesthetic. When the Stomach channel flow is suddenly switched from the correct direction to the backwards direction, the Stomach itself stops receiving electrical support for normal (downward) peristalsis (gut movement). When a person's stomach ceases to receive electrical instruction, the person may experience a decrease in appetite. In a case of severe shock or anesthesia, the person may automatically eject any food that might be in the stomach.

People with Parkinson's disease, whose Stomach channel flow has gradually, over decades, been altered, do not necessarily have constant, low-grade nausea, though some of my patients have had this symptom. However, many people with Parkinson's *do* have diminished appetites and often have trouble maintaining a healthy weight.

A. Calcaneus
B. Talus
C. Navicular
D. Cuboid
E. Medial (1st) Cuneiform
F. Intermediate (2nd) Cuneiform
G. Lateral (3rd) Cuneiform
H. 1st Metatarsal
I. 2nd Metatarsal
J. 3rd Metatarsal
K. 4th Metatarsal
L. 5th Metatarsal
M. 1st Phalange 1st toe
N. 1st Phalange 2nd toe
O. 1st Phalange 3rd toe
P. 1st Phalange 4th toe
Q. 1st Phalange 5th toe
R. 2nd Phalanges

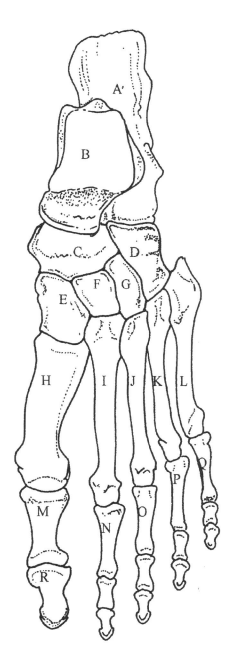

Fig. 12.1
The bones of the foot.

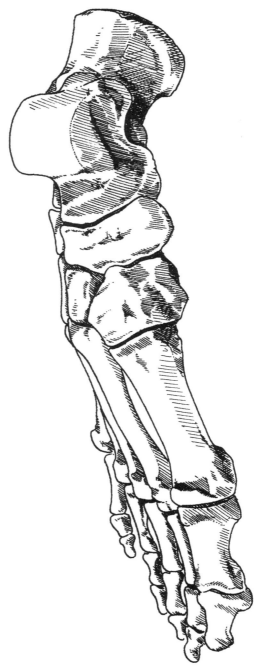

Fig. 12.2
Position 1: Medial-side view of the foot

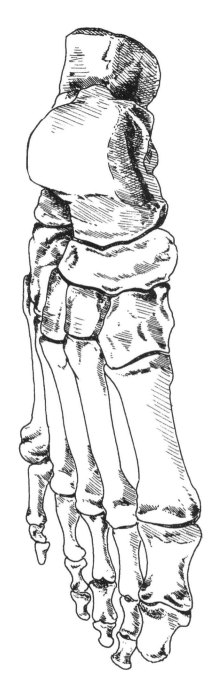

Fig. 12.3
Position 2: Foot rotating slightly medially

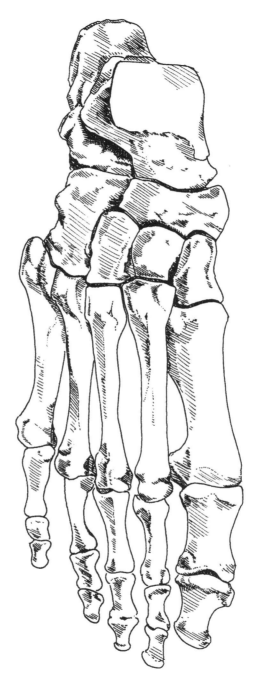

Fig. 12.4
Position 3: Top view of the foot

80

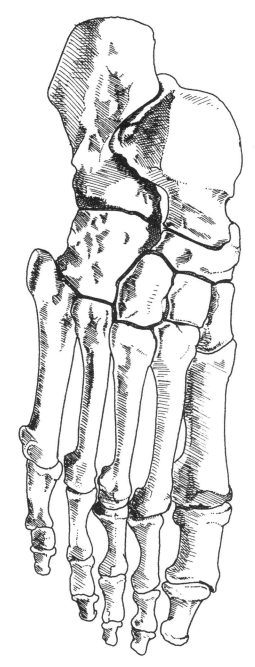

Fig. 12.5
Position 4: Continuing rotation

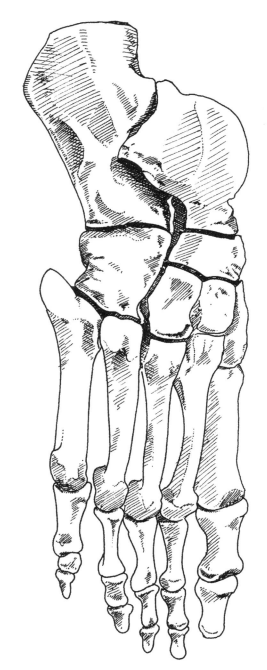

Fig. 12.5
Position 5: Continuing rotation

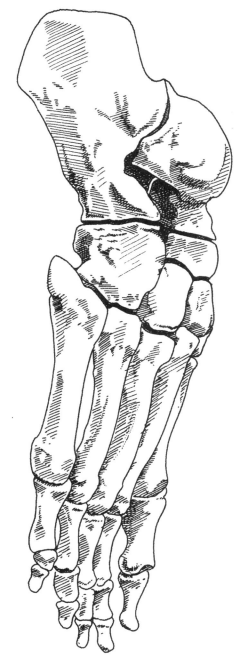

Fig. 12.7
Position 6: Lateral-side view of the foot

83

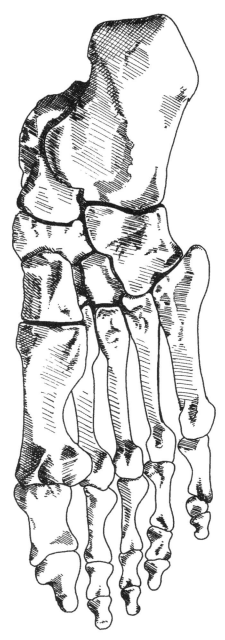

Fig. 12.8
Plantar view (looking at the bottom of the foot). Note the thin sliver of the intermediate cuneiform bone, nestled in between the 1st cuneiform and the 3rd cuneiform.

Suggestions for where to place your hands on the feet

After you've quickly, or slowly, worked your way down the leg from the relatively more responsive areas at the knee or hip and noticed how the areas responded or not, or want more work, you will end up at the ankles and feet.

It was relatively easy to describe "where to put the hands" when working on the arms and legs – place one hand on any side of the arm or leg and then place your other hand opposite the first one.

When it comes to the ankles and feet, it becomes much harder to *explain* exactly where the hands might want to go. Even so, within a few hours of practicing, it may become obvious – your hands will know what to do, even if your mind does not. But in the beginning it will seem easier to you if you have a few suggestions of where to place your hands.

Then again, I am almost hesitant to describe where, exactly, to place the hands when you've moved all the way down the leg to the ankle; many students cling too rigidly to whatever I write, particularly when I describe some ankle and foot holds, even though I state over and over that the following are just suggestions. But some people are so unaccustomed to holding feet and ankles that they truly do not know where to start. This chapter provides the suggestions for places that a practitioner can hold his hands. As you become more accustomed to holding and feeling, you will soon learn where to place your hands to give 1) firm support and 2) be comfortable.

The following list of possible places that you might want to put your hands also includes suggestions for directions in which you will perform your extremely gentle nudge, if any.

Again, the only reason for resting or nudging one's hands in these suggested positions is to determine whether or not the touch evokes a healthy response. You are *not* trying to forcefully move any bones, force looseness upon anything that feels tight, or force a displaced bone to its correct position.

The following suggestions will help you assess which areas might need more holding and if they need a different type of holding. If the areas do not respond to holding or nudging, they may be needing the "just sitting there, holding" variant of FSR that we use on people with Parkinson's or on anyone with a stubborn injury.

If you want to place your hands in different places than the ones suggested, do so. The following suggestions are merely to get you started.

Ankle and foot holding/nudging positions: some suggestions

Place a hand on either side of the ankle, with the medial and lateral malleoli (inner and outer ankle bones) each held snugly in a palm of your hand. If the ankle area feels responsive to your touch, good: you can move on. If not, make a note of it and move on, though you may wish to return to this area later.

Next, to find out about the ankle articulations, you may want to try nudging – or thinking about nudging (usually more effective) – the ankle bones in a few different planes of movement.

Try not to dwell on how you think the ankles *should* move. Just notice that the ankles move or don't when you firmly hold or gently nudge them in.

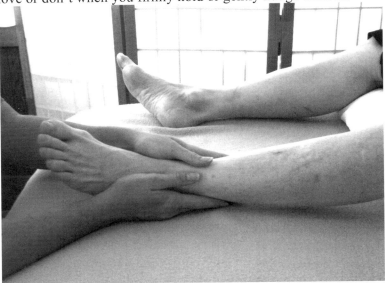

Fig. 12.9   Holding the ankles

You may wish to push your hands that are holding the ankle bones towards each other and note if the ankles respond by moving in the opposite (outward) direction. You may wish to see if the ankle bones will nestle closer to each other as a rebound move when you imagine that your hands, closely connected to the skin of the ankle bones, move slightly apart for a moment. Moving your hands apart is the opposite of nudging them together.

You may also want to try mentally moving your hand in such a way as if one of the ankle bones, for a fleeting moment, would be nudged upwards, towards the thigh, while the other one moves downward, towards the heel. See if there is any sign of a response. If not, make a note of it. If there was no response, you may want to return to this area later. If there was a response, you still might want to keep holding the ankle so see if there is a response when you think about moving your hands forwards and backwards relative to each other, and then the reverse.

The main thing you will want to do is practice doing simple holding or maybe directional nudgings on many healthy feet so that you can ascertain just how a normal set of ankle bones moves in relation to the leg bones, the heel bone, the talus bone, and each other. Even if you don't know how all these bones should move in theory, if you hold enough feet and try minutely or mentally nudging your hands over most of the areas of the feet, you will soon come to have a sense of what a foot should feet like, and how it should respond to being held.

When you've finished assessing/holding the ankles bones, you might want to move on to the heel.

86

Holding the heel bone

One way to hold the heel bone is one hand under the calcaneus (heel bone), holding that round ball of the heel cupped in one hand, with the other hand supporting the Achilles tendon from behind.

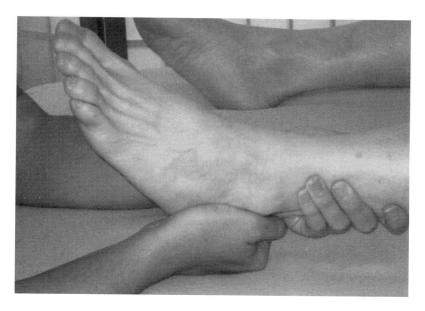

Fig. 12.10 Holding the heel and the Achilles tendon

Notice: are you holding a healthy, responsive ankle/tendon? If yes, then good. But if nothing seems to be moving, or this intersection of the Achilles tendon and the heel bone seems uncannily rigid, you may want to gently and quickly nudge or imagine a nudge as you bring your hands together and then let your hands rebound back into position.

In this case, your hands will be bringing the calcaneus a bit closer to the Achilles tendon. Or you might think of it as bringing the tendon closer to the calcaneus. It doesn't matter. The main thing is to notice if there's any sort of response.

As before, if a gentle nudge gets no response, wait half a minute or so and try a the merest of mental nudges. If still nothing happens, wait half a minute and try a slightly stronger nudge.

Also consider moving your right hand posteriorly (towards the back) while your left hand moves anteriorly (towards the front). And then try the reverse, right hand anteriorly and left hand posteriorly.

And what happens if you nudge, or mentally nudge one hand to the left and the other to the right, and then the reverse? Learn how healthy feet respond to this sort of play, and then, when you hold your patient's injured foot, you will have a sense as to whether or not all is well in this area.

If all is well in the ankle, a movement or thought that *compresses* the joining of the calcaneus and Achilles tendon, bringing them closer together, should evoke a rebounding apart in the ankle after you are done nudging. Oppositely, a nudge that suggests microscopically pulling the tendon/calcaneous junction *apart* should evoke a tiny coming-together response in the two parts. In either case, the area should respond.

Immediately or eventually, in response to your holding or nudging, the heel bone/Achilles relationship may feel responsive. If it does, good. If not, make a note to yourself that this area might want some deeper work at a later date and then move on.

On the other hand, you may feel that slightly nudging (or thinking about nudging) the heel sideways to the left while thinking about moving the tendon to the right (or vice versa) one more time would be a good thing to do. Fine. Do it. Possibly by getting the heel/tendon relationship to loosen up by moving from side to side, the relationship will also loosen up in other directions as well. Do what you like, do what your intuition tells you to do, do what the patient's ankle tells you to do. Let go of the ankle if the patient's ankle tells you to Let go.

Try some or all of these suggestions on healthy feet so that you can learn to understand how this tendon/heel relationship works when everything is moving nicely.

The Talus-Calcaneus relationship

Next, if you are satisfied that the heel/tendon was moving properly, or you decided that it wasn't and you made a mental note to return there later on, you might wish to place one hand on the talus bone and the other behind the back corner of the calcaneous (heel bone). Or you may wish to choose some other area to hold. These are just suggestions.

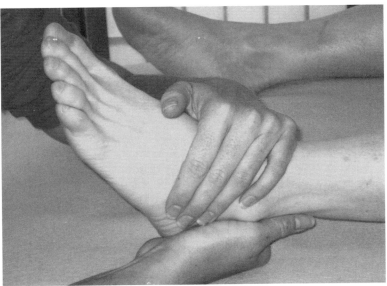

Fig. 12.11 Holding the talus and calcaneus bones

Do the usual routine on these bones to assess whether or not they can move. The "usual routine" means that you will notice if the foot feels responsive when you support these bones. If not, then you will gently nudge these bones towards each other. Or possibly, you will gently imagine them moving apart. Or you might nudge them or imagine them moving one to the left, the other to the right. Or you might think that one is moving towards the head and the other is moving towards the toes. You can try to test these bones on any directional plane that you can imagine.

When you work on a healthy foot by gently provoking a reflexive response in every possible direction you will be able to develop an innate sense of the way that these bones can and should move, relative to each other.

An aside: foot bones might make very small movements

Do bear in mind that even if these bones can move correctly, they may not move very far. They *may* jerk around if they've been significantly displaced, but it's more likely that they may move just a *tiny* bit, making a barely perceptible response. Of course, there is always the possibility that they will make a generous sweeping relaxation movement. But you should have no expectation, one way or the other.

Your hands, only through experience, can eventually know what it feels like to work with a responsive foot. The movements, tiny or languorous, that do occur will feel "right" to you if they are right. If you do the nudging and the imagined nudging and nothing happens, if you do the tiny pushes and pulsing and you get a sense that the bones involved are putting their backs up and saying, "No!" then you will know that, possibly, this is an area that maybe wants some simple, boring holding: support, support, support.

Don't try to change its mind; just make a note that this area wants more work and go on to the next place. Or stay here and hold, just supporting, with no significant moving, for a long time.

Navicular-Calcaneus relationship

Next, you may wish to place one hand on the navicular bone and the other behind the back corner (heel) of the calcaneous. Again, determine whether or not this area can respond.

Or you may wish to put one hand on the navicular bone and the other on the talus. Or you may want to drape the middle finger of one hand over the navicular bone with the thumb of the same hand supporting the sole of the foot. (Photo on next page.)

Or possibly, you will find that placing your thumb over the talus and the rest of the hand around the back of the ankle may feel the best for you.

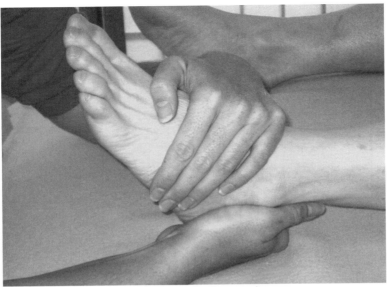
Fig. 12.12 Holding the navicular and calcaneus bones

If this part of the foot doesn't relax in response to supportive holding, you may try gently pulsing your hands together in such a way that the navicular and talus bones are pressed towards each other. Or you might try thinking about your hands pulling apart from each other. Or move one of your hands that's over a bone to the left, and the other hand to the right, or move one of them towards the front of the foot and the other towards the back.

An aside: working with less than a full hand

The curves of the foot are often so small that it is impossible to place the entire hand over some foot part. For example, when supportively holding the big toe, sometimes you can only fit a little bit of your hand around the toe, or maybe you can only fit one finger up against one side of the toe and another finger on the other side of the toe.

Likewise, because of the curve of the foot's arch, it may be impossible to place the whole palm of your hand firmly up against the bottom of the foot. In this case, instead of using your palm, you can nestle the gently curved *backside* of your hand up against the sole of the arch. In other words, the important thing here is the supportive contact, not which part of your hand or how *much* of your hand you are using to provide the support. For that matter, sometimes when I am working on a patient's foot and I sense that the patient would feel more supported if I had a third hand, I press my shoulder gently up against some part of the sole of the patient's foot while I am using both hands to support the ankle.

I am so short that, sitting on a stool at the foot of the treatment table, the table comes up to the middle of my chest. My shoulder is only a few inches higher. If the patient's foot is close enough to the edge of the treatment table, I can lean forward, causing the patient's foot to press up against my shoulder, thus using my shoulder as a third hand.

90

I am not saying that you need to do this. What I am trying to get across is that the patient must feel supported by human touch, and it is your job as practitioner to provide the support. A supportive pillow is not the same as a human hand. But sometimes, that "human hand" doesn't need to be the full palm of the hand, or even a hand, per se. A mere finger or a shoulder can sometimes serve the function of a hand.

If your palm doesn't fit comfortably onto the area that you are working on, use whatever part of your hand does fit, so that you can provide support, support, support.

Cuboid bone

Place the palms of one hand over the top (dorsum) and the palm of the other hand over the bottom (sole) of the cuboid bone. Look for a response.

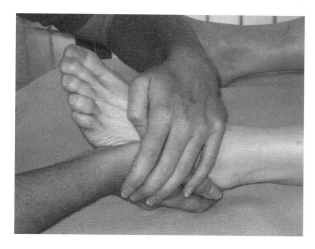

Fig. 12.13 Holding the cuboid bone

And/or place one hand on the lateral side of the cuboid bone. With the other hand, grip the navicular bone between the thumb and middle finger. If there is no response, quickly and gently compress the bones towards each other and release.

Or hold it any way you like. Be comfortable.

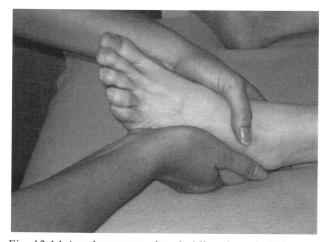

Fig. 12.14 Another approach to holding the cuboid bone

The cuneiforms

Place the palm of each hand on either side (sole and top of the foot) of the medial cuneiform. If no response, compress (nudge) and release. Hold until you feel a relaxation response.

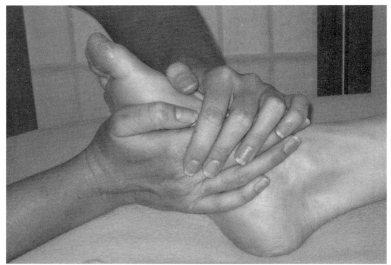
Fig. 12.15 Holding the medial cuneiform bone

Place the palms of the hands on either side of the intermediate cuneiform bone. If no response, compress and release. Hold until you feel a relaxation response.

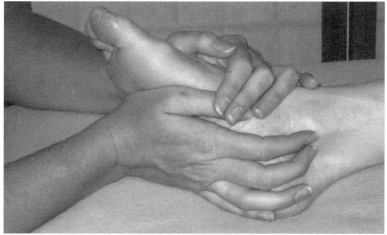
Fig. 12.16   Holding the intermediate cuneiform bone

Somewhere between your first and your hundredth treatment on a given person with Parkinson's, this bone may shudder or jerk or possibly even whip around. Until then, just do all the above supportive holdings and note whether or not the area is capable of

92

responding. As always, if it can't respond, make a mental note of this and plan on simply holding in this area for a long time.

On the other hand, if the intermediate cuneiform bone falls back into place, the cuboid or some other bone(s) might suddenly slide back into position, as well! In that case, the next time you revisit the cuboid bone it will be setting nicely, and perfectly responsive, even though you haven't yet worked on it directly. The first time your work on a Parkinson's patient, this area probably will *not* be responsive.

Lateral, also known as 3rd, cuneiform bone

Place the palms of the hands on either side of the lateral cuneiform bone: one hand on top of the foot, the other hand on the bottom (sole) of the foot. As mentioned before, if it feels stodgy or stubborn, try gently nudging your hands towards each other to see if the foot tissues between your hands will push back outward on your hands.

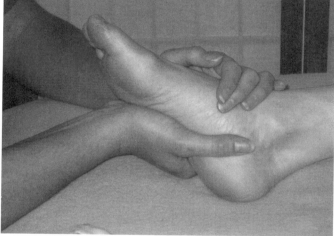

Fig. 12.17   Holding the lateral cuneiform bone

All three cuneiforms at once

Place your palm or the middle fingers of both hands over either side (top and sole) of the cuneiform bones as a group. Compress and release, (nudge) either physically or in your imagination.

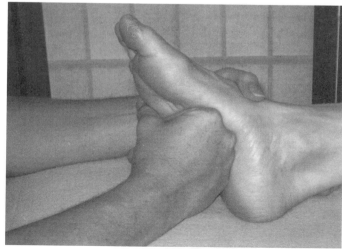

Fig. 12.18 Holding all three cuneiforms at once

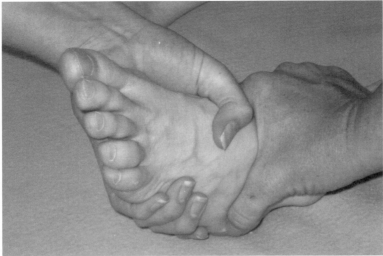

Fig. 12.19 Holding all three cuneiforms at once – another approach

Or you might grip the cuneiform bones with one hand (thumb and middle finger over the top and sole) and grip the navicular bone with the other hand (top and sole). Nudge the cuneiform bones, as a group, towards the navicular bone and release – or towards the metacarpals and release.

Metatarsals: the long skinny bones of the feet

Place a hand on either side (top and sole) of the proximal (closer to the torso, farther from the tips of the toes) end of the 1st metatarsal. Compress your hands towards each other and release. Move the hand so that the center of your palm is centered over the 2nd metatarsal and repeat. Repeat in this manner over the proximal ends of all 5 metatarsals.

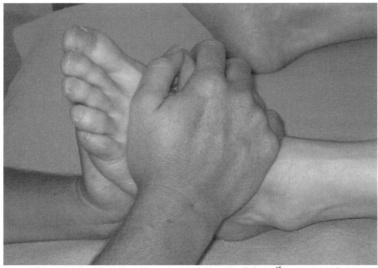

Fig. 12.20   Holding the proximal end of the 1st metatarsal

Place the palm of either hand over either side (top and sole) of the *distal* (farther from the torso, closer to the tips of the toes) end of the 1st metatarsal. If no relaxation response, compress and release. Repeat for all 5 metatarsals.

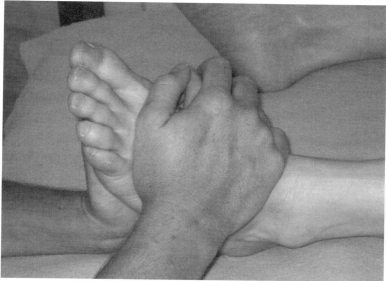

Fig. 12.21   Holding the distal end of the 3rd metatarsal

Metatarsal- cuneiform joints

Grip the cuneiforms with the thumb and middle finger over the top and sole. With the thumb on one side and index and middle finger on the other, grip the proximal end of the 1st metatarsal. Compress the metatarsal towards the nearest cuneiform and release. Repeat this with the other 4 metatarsals.

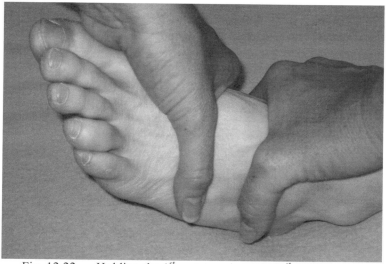

Fig. 12.22   Holding the 1st metatarsal and the 1st cuneiform

Toes

Place thumb and index (or middle, or fourth) finger on either side (top and sole) of the first phalange of the big toe. Compress and release.

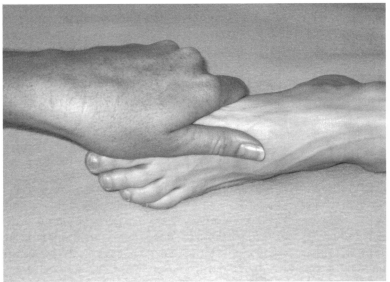

Fig. 12.23   Holding the 1st (the big) toe

Move to the first phalange of the second toe. Compress and release. Repeat across all five toes.

Move to the second phalange of the big toe. Compress and release. Repeat across all toes until all the phalanges have been relaxed.

Note: The toe joints may move very quickly, and the movements, if any, are usually *very* small. I usually only spend a few seconds assessing each toe unless there is something clearly wrong in a toe joint. If there is a problem with a specific toe, then spend extra time and attention on that one spot. In general, the toes will be responsive and will not even require much holding.

Hammertoes and other toe contortions are very often caused by tensions a *good distance away* from the toes: the problem may be coming from the cuneiforms, the ankle joints or even the legs. Some of the worst hammertoes I've ever seen have been resolved by working on the ankles or legs – not on the toes.

Sometimes hammertoes relax in response to work done on the *center* of the foot: sometimes hammertoes don't relax until the *ankles* relax. I've *never* seen them relax due to working on the toes themselves.

Repeat the above toe sequence with the thumb and finger-of-choice on either side (medial and lateral) of each toe, going over every phalange.

You can go over the whole foot many times. It may be that every time you go over it, microscopic movements will take place, leading up to restoring of the correct articulations after many seemingly "no response" treatments.

You can hold the bones in the ankle-to-toes sequential order suggested above or in whatever order you feel like, several times. If some stubbornly held place does release in response to your holding, it is very likely that some other previously stuck joint articulation may also now be able to move.

The bones are assembled somewhat like those old wooden ball puzzles in which the pieces are so curiously interconnected that you cannot really move any puzzle piece until you figure out which one to move first. Sometimes it may seem as if no bones will move until they are *all* ready to move. On each pass over the foot, each bone may make scarcely perceptible adjustments even when you are doing nothing but quickly assessing. At some point, all of the bones may have corrected their own positions enough so that suddenly they will *all* move smoothly and easily into their correct position.

On the other hand, while working your way across the foot and ankle, it is very likely that you will come across one or several locations that feature such supreme rigidity that you can safely assume that this area wants something deeper.

This area probably wants the resting-in-one-place-for-a-long-time type of holding: the FSR that we do on stubborn or complex injuries.

Finish going over the foot, making your assessments, and then, returning to the place that seemed to want the most work, sit back, get comfortable, and apply the "no motion, no nudging, no intention" type of FSR in the location that needs it. Or, if you prefer, you may stop the assessment process when you find an "obvious" place that needs holding, and settle in.

Which shall it be? Stop exploring and just hold the place where you detect a stubborn problem, or keep going and come back to it later? You decide. Follow your intuition.

Neither sequence nor timing for "correct" FSR is carved in stone

You truly can approach the sequence and timing of the leg-to-foot FSR in whatever manner seems best to you, according to the silent instructions that you are receiving from your patient's leg and foot.

The most frequent remarks from health practitioners who came to Santa Cruz in order to observe members of the Parkinson's Treatment Research Team (1998 – 2013) doing FSR can be paraphrased this way: "I think I'm starting to get it; I've seen five of you doing FSR, and you're all doing exactly the same thing, namely nothing but sitting there holding the patient's foot, but you're all doing it so differently! And when I watched one of you in particular working on the same patient that you'd worked on a week earlier, you approached his leg and foot completely differently the second time."

A teaching video: an aside

Although many people have asked for a video or DVD of someone practicing the holding techniques illustrated in this chapter, it would be pointless: there is nothing to see. A video of me holding someone's ankle to see if there was a subtle responsiveness would just show, to the observer, footage of me sitting motionless, with my hands motionless, on a person's motionless ankle. I might sit there for several minutes or an hour, not doing anything, waiting for the ankle to respond. This would be supremely boring.

Again, there would *probably* be nothing to see.

Years ago, I gave in to popular demand and made a video of myself holding a person's leg, ankle, and foot in various holding positions. I spoke into the microphone very clearly, stating that I was *not* actually doing FSR. FSR is very slow and boring to watch. Instead, I was merely placing my hands on the subject's leg, ankle and foot in order to demonstrate some of the possible holds that a person might want to try. I moved fairly quickly through the various hand poses, stating over and over that I was just demonstrating a sampling of hand positions in order to help people get started who might otherwise be shy about putting their hands on someone's foot; I was *not* actually doing FSR.

After I released the video, I got many complaints from patients: previous to seeing the video, their therapists, working only from my book, had been going nice and slow, feeling their way along the legs and feet of their patients, spending as much time at each location as was necessary to bring about relaxation.

But *after* seeing the video, the therapists had copied the *tempo* of my videoed hand movements. Just as I had quickly moved from one position to another, the therapists were now moving their hands quickly from one spot to another. The *visual* cues from the video were too compelling; the spoken instructions on the video were completely ignored.

If I ever release another video, it will be the most boring thing on earth. In it, I shall demonstrate the tempo at which I go when a person's legs do not respond at all: I shall set my hands down in one place and hold them there for a solid minute or two, maybe half an hour. Any nudging or movement on my part would, correctly, be so small as to be invisible.

Then I will go to the next holding position and hold my hands there for half an hour. It will take an hour before the viewer has seen the merest fraction of all the possible ways that a practitioner might want to set his hands down on his patient. It will be so boring, no one will watch more than a few minutes of it before he is saying, "Enough already! Just show me the various hand positions, I understand that I am supposed to go slowly."

But I will not be fooled this time into thinking that this attempt will be different: too many people will *not* understand. Also, every patient is different. Each patient might need to have his foot bones held from a slightly different position and for a different amount of time.

People usually follow visual images more exactly than they follow words. The whole point of FSR is that the practitioner has to learn to follow his hunches and respond to the patient, not to a video. So I suspect that there will not be another foot-holding video in my future.

The next group of photos are merely for review: they show more of the basic hand positions for holding the intermediate cuneiform bone – a place where you will probably spend most of your time if you are treating a person with Parkinson's or a person with a mid-foot injury.

Three pictures: basic foot holding positions with focus on the cuneiform bones

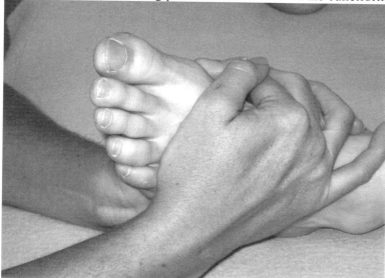

Fig 12.24   Holding the intermediate cuneiform

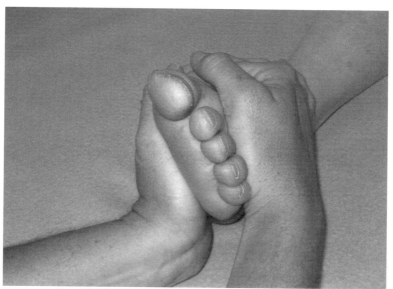

Fig. 12.25   Holding the intermediate cuneiform

The palm of the hand is flush on the sole of the foot, same as the previous photo, but viewed from a different angle.

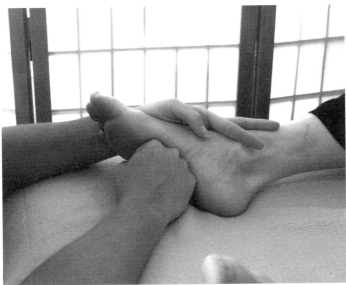

Fig. 12.26   Holding the cuneiform: the back of the hand is flush against the sole of the foot

As you can see, either the palm or the back of the hand can be used. It makes no difference. The important thing is to be able to give a feeling of complete, full support to the bottom and top of the foot.

This chapter has shown many examples of ways that you can hold someone's foot. Please do not think that you must place your hands in any or all or the positions shown above. It is better to just place your hands where they feel like they are supporting whatever area seems to need support, based on that area's inability to relax and be responsive.

An example of a difficult hand placement

I once treated a patient who had impaled his foot on a pitchfork. The fork entered his foot from the front, slicing in between the first and second toe and drove in deeply to the center of the foot. The injury had occurred many years earlier but the white scar was still quite visible between the toes. There was no way I could place my entire hand between his toes. Instead, I wiggled my index finger into the space between the first and second toe. My other three fingers looped around the bottom of the ball of the foot and came to rest on the medial (inside) side of the big toe. My thumb pointed towards my index finger and was somewhat wedged into the groove that runs between the toes and the sole of the foot, under the three lateral toes. My other hand was holding his ankle. I just sat like that for the full hour, giving very firm support to the area with the pitchfork scar. After several weeks of holding just like this, during a holding session, the entire foot relaxed, all the toes, especially the first and second, separated wide apart, and the patient reported feeling warmth and life spreading throughout his foot.

This example is provided to show that it is not always necessary to get the whole hand onto an injured spot. I was using only my index finger on the spot indicated. But the whole rest of my right hand was also providing support, and my left hand was bringing up the rear by supporting the *ankle* against the pressure being applied from the front end of the foot.

An important aside

Before the publication of this book, a much shorter, five-chapter leaflet, *FSR for Parkinson's*, was available for free, online. These chapters had no photographs whatsoever – only text descriptions of the basic concepts, short descriptions of some possible hand positions, and a few pen and ink drawings of holding the forearm.

Working from these simple text descriptions, having no photos to "follow," many people with no bodywork experience whatsoever were able to master the FSR enough so that their Parkinson's patient recovered. It is simple, supportive holding, such as anyone might intuitively do for any injured person, *if* they had not learned the cultural restrictions that make us afraid of touching. Holding an injured person is *not* rocket science.

The following was excerpted from an email from someone I've never met. She was working from the photo-less, short-version instructions in *FSR for Parkinson's*. She was treating her husband who had Parkinson's disease. It demonstrates my point:

"Thank you. I am sitting here crying with relief. I don't want to inundate you with emails but I think you may be interested in what happened last night. I have lacked confidence in my ability to hold my husband's foot properly and in the end I just had to trust, although I had not been doing very much. The last two nights I have spent about an hour holding, sometimes falling asleep while I am doing it. Last night I got the usual tingling sensation in my hands but stronger and having worked my way down his leg I was holding his foot. (He has been telling me that he had experienced leg twitching after one holding session so I took that as a good sign.)

"Last night when I reached his foot the sensation was very strong. I saw in my mind an ice blue light in his foot and then he literally leaped off the bed as if he had been given an electric shock. He did not wake up.

"I didn't say anything to him because I did not want to influence any response and he told me, unprompted, that he felt looser and more flexible. Then I told him what had happened. His face looked more healthy to me this morning and he adjusted his posture to something so close to normal. The angle of his head and neck was a miracle to see.

"…Thank you… We will continue on our own for now but I don't feel alone or unsupported anymore…"

This person was obviously doing a great job of holding her spouse's foot. She was not working from photographs, or any visual cues. She was not sure of herself. But she just started holding his foot. Eventually, his foot, and then his body, came back to life.

So don't follow the photos too closely. They are just suggestions. At some point, within the first session or the second, you should put this book aside and stop thinking about "technique" and just enjoy yourself. The most important thing to remember is support, support, support.

Support, support, support.

Chapter thirteen

Testing the feet

Apply some tests! While a foot's increased ability to move in the directions described in this chapter is not a 100% guarantee that displacements or electrical blockages are completely gone, it can be a fairly good indication that things are going the right way.

A healthy reflex

The foot has a wonderful reflex that it can do only when all of the bones in the foot are gliding across their articulations freely and easily. The reflex can be triggered with the following stimulation:

The patient should be lying down on a treatment table with straight legs. Place one hand over the patient's foot, with the center of the palm placed on the top, or dorsum of the foot, directly *over* the intermediate cuneiform bone. The rest of the hand can rest on the top of the foot wherever it's comfortable. Then, place your other hand, in a fist position, on the *sole* of the foot, *under* the intermediate cuneiform bone.

Press the hands together slightly and then release. This use of the word "press" refers to an actual, physical compression, one that's visible to the naked eye. The press should be almost instantly be followed by relaxation back to the starting position.

This pressing and relaxing is a *significant* movement, as opposed to the mental, infinitesimally small nudges and pulsing movements that you've used up until now. You are doing this to initiate a reflex muscle movement in the foot.

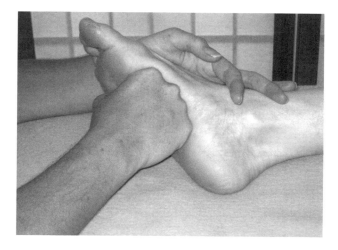

Fig.13.1 Quickly pressing a bit hard, looking for a reflexive movement

Your hands should remain on the foot during the subsequent reflexive movement, if any. The foot, if its bones are all in the correct position and unhampered by tensions *might*, in response to being very gently punched on the sole of the foot, reflexively relax in one of two directions. The two reflexive foot movements are these:

1.   The foot may stretch out as if the toes are being pointed like a ballerina. The center line of the top of the foot will straighten out, forming a straight line which is a continuation of the tibial crest (the bony front ridge of the lower-leg bone). (Fig. 13.2)

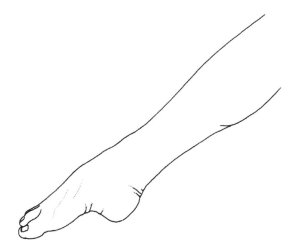

Fig. 13.2   A straight line from leg to toes

A completely relaxed foot, when pushed quickly and gently in the arch area, might easily go into a pointed-toe position. If the ankle is *also* aligned correctly, the ridge of the tibial crest to the center of the foot will form a nice, almost straight line. If there is a problem in the ankle area, the ankle joint may form a concave dip instead of making a nice smooth line.

When the foot injury fully heals, your patient will be able to form this pointed toe posture on his own, without needing to be pushed in the arch.

2.   The foot may rotate, causing the toes to form a line that is perpendicular to the floor. The big toe will be the toe which is farthest from the surface of the table. The line from the big toe through the little toe forms the perpendicular line. (See Fig. 13.4.)

In the starting position, the right foot is pointing towards the ceiling, and midline of the right foot is more or less in a straight line with the knee.

In the following drawing (Fig 13.3), the right foot appears to be pointing forward more than the left foot. This is because the right foot has been held for a bit, and has become more relaxed than the left foot.

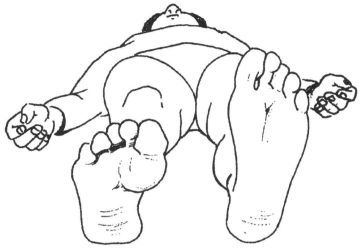

Fig 13.3 Relaxed foot, after FSR

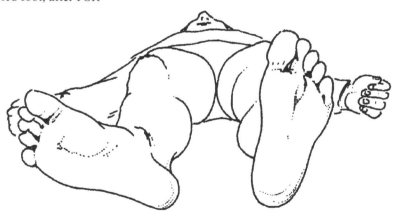

Fig. 13.4   Foot rotation in response to a push on the arch

After being bumped gently but firmly in the arch, the right foot may respond, if it is completely relaxed and flexible, by rotating laterally (out to the side, Fig. 13.4, above). The knee will *not* have rotated a considerable distance; the rotation will have come from mostly from the relaxed ankle.

If the foot articulations are not yet correct, the response to the reflex test may be:
1. The foot will not straighten out as in fig. 13.2, but will instead remain at more or less of a right angle to the tibia (main bone of the lower leg): the original position.
2. Instead of rotating laterally as in fig. 13.4, a foot that is still injured may reflexively rotate medially, *towards* the side with the arch, as if protecting the arch of the foot instead of exposing it.

Hammer-toes

Also, if displacements or unhealed injuries are present in the foot, ankle and/or leg, the over-taut tendons in these areas may pull back on the toes, creating hammer-toes (see Fig.s 13.5 and 13.6).

Hammer-toes are not uncommon. Hammer-toes do *not* mean a person is at risk for Parkinson's disease. That having been said, hammer-toes are a sure sign that there is tension or injury somewhere in the foot, ankle, lower leg, knee, or even somewhere upstream from the knee.

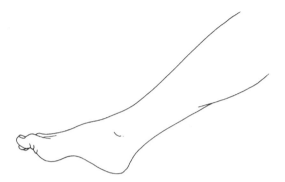

Fig. 13.5   Moderate hammer-toe of the first (big) toe

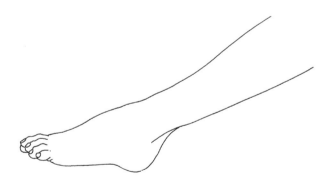

Fig 13.6   Mild hammer-toe of the second toe

If a hammer-toe is present, your work *might* not be done. The presence of a hammer-toe suggests that the foot is still not fully relaxed. However, patients have recovered from problematic foot injuries and from Parkinson's even though their hammer-toes never went away. If your patient has recovered normal foot flexibility and no longer has pain, or if his Parkinson's symptoms are going away don't worry about the hammer-toe.

I have had PD patients with severe hammer-toes who recovered from Parkinson's even with some residual amount of hammer-toe. Still, some recovered patients worry about their hammer toes so I repeat: if your patient has recovered from PD but still has some hammer-toe, don't worry about it. Leave it be. Or work on it if your patient wants you to.

Don't be pushy

Be very careful when you do test the feet to insure that *you are not trying to exert influence over the direction of the foot reflex*.

Do your quick push on the arch and then be a passive observer of which way the foot wants to go. Sometimes it is hard to be impartial; after working for hours on a foot, it is only natural that you will be secretly rooting for the foot to relax straight and long and/or rotate outward. But try not to impose your wishes on that foot. Do a realistic assessment of the reflex. When the foot responds correctly to this test, and the joints all seem to glide smoothly and easily, and there are no areas of the foot that feel somehow less than "correct," you *may* be finished with working on the feet. If so, congratulations.

Flexible feet that still want FSR

You may not yet be finished working on the feet. You are finished when the patient can move his feet normally in all the usual directions, he can *feel* his foot moving, he *likes* the feeling of moving his foot, and there is no pain in his foot.

Sometimes, because of residual *emotional* resistance in the injured area, you may not be finished with FSR on the foot in question – even if *you* can move the foot around easily.

Because slow and steady FSR can be an effective way to assist in emotional healing, as well as structural healing, sometimes FSR will still be beneficial even after the foot begins to resume flexibility.

A common question is "How will I know when the foot no longer needs to be held."

Answers:

If *you* can move the patient's foot easily in all the normal directions, but the patient can't move his own feet easily, at will, continue with foot FSR treatments and encourage your patient to continue doing the light and energy exercise in chapter five.

If the foot relaxes *sometimes*, but tightens up at other times, the patient is using pause or intermittently dissociating from foot during those times when the foot it tight.

A physical injury does *not* come and go. The use of self-induced dissociation or pause can come and go, depending on how the person has instilled his self-protection instructions. In the case of self-induced protection, rigidity in the legs and feet might be able to come and go, based on mood or other circumstances.

Again, if the foot is sometimes relaxed and sometimes rigid, it is the patient's thoughts and not an injury that is causing the change ups. FSR will *not* help with this. The patient must get rid of his self-created protection behaviors, whether dissociation or pause.

In Chinese medicine, the difference between a problem that comes and goes is differentiated from a problem that is constant, with a fixed location. The come-and-go problem is considered to be a mentally-instigated (though usually subconscious) channel Qi blocking problem referred to as "Qi Stagnation." You might think of this in English as an energy-*directing* problem.

Oppositely, a constant, unchanging problem in a fixed location is referred to in Chinese medicine as "Blood Stagnation." Blood stagnation usually comes from some tangible damage or injury.

If foot rigidity or blockage of energy in the foot comes and goes, the underlying problem is coming from the mind of the patient.

If the person has been diagnosed with Parkinson's disease, it is most *likely* that the patient is using self-induced pause. As noted quite a few times already, pause should be terminated before using any type of Yin Tui Na.

Chapter fourteen

Shoulders and hips

Shoulder and hip injuries and displacements are not unusual. Sometimes the patient will know the exact location of the problem, but often, you will need to find the exact location of the injury by looking for an area that doesn't relax in response to being held.

If the injury seems to be in a *rotational* (ball and socket) joint such as the hip or the shoulder, there are a number of ways in which the joint might be held. This chapter will offer a few starter suggestions on ways to hold these more complex areas. Of course, once the practitioner is comfortable with working on rotational joints, he will allow his hands to take the lead in deciding where to be placed.

You will be looking for areas with underlying unhealed injuries if the patient has pain or unusual stiffness in some area, or if you have noticed some rigidity in an area that just doesn't feel right. If the patient remembers an injury, you will of course explore that area.

Many people with Parkinson's will have unhealed injuries in areas other than just the foot, including the shoulder and hip areas.

Shoulder

Have the patient lie on his back. Slide one of your hands under his scapula (shoulder blade).

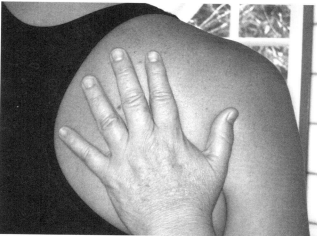

Fig. 14.1   A hand placed on the patient's scapula (shown with patient standing)

Rest your other hand firmly in the depression just below the shoulder edge of the clavicle, on the front side of the body – just above the lung. (Fig. 14.2)

With one hand firmly under the scapula, quickly press down firmly with the clavicle hand and then immediately let up on the pressure. If there is no injury and the joint is relaxable, the scapula will respond to this press by moving medially – towards the spine. If the shoulder area has an injury or is fearful, when you quickly compress-and-release the clavicle towards the scapula, the scapula will move laterally – away from the spine – as if trying to rotate around to the front of the body: curling forward as if to protect the injury.

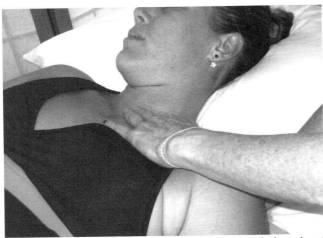

Fig. 14.2 The lower hand on the scapula, upper hand just below the clavicle

If the scapula doesn't move at all, that also suggests a protective, or even dissociated situation in the shoulder and/or overall body.

If the above test, or a visually obvious displacement of anything in the shoulder area, suggests an unhealed injury, consider the following hand positions for your FSR work.

The patient should be lying on his back. Seat yourself facing the patient, at about the level of the patient's shoulder

Place one hand, the hand closest to the person's head, around the "epaulet" area – where the arm inserts into the shoulder socket, and where the lateral end of the clavicle terminates. Get a good, firm grip on this rounded area. (Fig. 14.3)

Place the other hand on the center of the upper-arm bone, the humerus. The best way to position this other hand is to bring it *under* the arm, gripping the side of the humerus that is resting on the table, rather than gripping the humerus from the top (facing the ceiling) side. (Fig. 14.3)

With your hands in these two positions, one cupping the shoulder/ball of the arm-bone and the other firmly gripping the shaft of the humerus, the patient's shoulder joint will feel absolutely supported. Maybe waggle your hands a tiny bit, to show yourself and the patient just how firmly you are supporting the shoulder.

Now that you've got a good, supportive hold, gently nudge-and-release (so gently that the patient *cannot* feel it), or *imagine* nudging, the ball at the top of the humerus bone a bit deeper *into* the shoulder socket. Notice if there is a response. Very often, the response

110

will seem like the humerus moves away from the socket, in opposition to what you have suggested. So long as any movement response occurs, fine. Go on to the next nudge.

Very gently nudge the humerus as if you are pulling it slightly *out* of the socket. Again, note if a response occurs.

You will now do a series of twelve nudges that will check the responsiveness of all the various muscles and articulations that circle the shoulder. Imagine that a ring around the ball of the humerus is numbered one through twelve, like the face of an old fashioned clock.

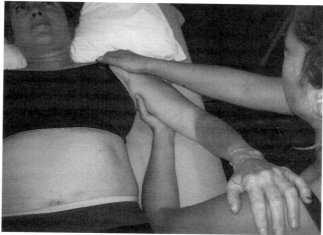

Fig. 14.3   One hand on the lateral top (epaulet area) of the shoulder, the other holding the humerus.

I usually imagine that the number one is located at the top humerus, just under the acromion (lateral end of the clavicle). The number six is at the bottom of the ball of the humerus, in the armpit. On the right arm, the three is located at the anterior (forward) side of the ball of the humerus, and the nine is located at the posterior (back) side of the ball. On the left arm, the three is posterior and the nine is anterior. This all sounds very fancy but, really, when you sit down and imagine a clock face, it becomes pretty simple and obvious.

The other numbers are placed sequentially around the ball of the humerus, like the numbers on a round (analog) clock face.

These numbers are mentally superimposed merely to help keep track of the small increments you will nudge in, as you work your way around the shoulder. Once you've mentally got your orienting numbers in place, briefly, *imperceptibly* nudge the humerus upwards, towards the number one and then immediately relax back to your original position. Notice if there was *any* tiny reaction or movement in the area in response to the nudge.

If *so*, go on to the number two and give the arm bone a nudge in that direction. If *not*, do *increasingly* subtle nudges in the direction of the number one. If, after several nudges, including one that is purely imaginary, nothing moves, make a mental note to return to this area, and move on to number two, where you repeat the assessment process. And so on, around the "clock."

After making the rounds of the "clock," return to any area that simply refused to respond and settle in for a good long sit, with your hands supporting the shoulder area: one hand cupped over the shoulder and the other hand firmly gripping the humerus. Now and then, as inspired to do so, try again to give an imperceptible nudge in the direction that was frozen. And now and then, place the hands in the first shoulder testing position, with one hand under the scapula and the other hand in the depression just below the clavicle.

These hand-position suggestions will give you a start at feeling comfortable with "where to put the hands" while working on the shoulder. As you get more familiar with the sensation of working with the shoulder joint, you can feel free to try other holding positions, as well. You should first try this on a person with healthy shoulders. It is very common to find hang-ups, that is to say, areas that won't budge, on healthy people who have had a dislocated shoulder, broken arms, falls from a bicycle, or other arm/shoulder injuries. So do not be discouraged if your practice partner turns out to have some areas that don't move. Be pleased! You can go ahead and treat the asymptomatic person, thus preventing a possible painful shoulder situation that might have otherwise crept up in old age.

Hip and leg joint

The hip area is very similar to the shoulder area: the ball of the femur (the femur is the long bone of the upper leg) rotates in the hip socket in very much the same manner that the ball of the humerus rotates in the shoulder socket.

Sit or stand facing the patient, just below the level of the hip. Place one hand under the lateral-distal (lateral means closer to the side, or your might say farther from the spine; distal means closer to the feet, farther from the head) part of the buttock. Elevate the patient's near knee while keeping his near foot flat on the table. Next, using your other arm, bend your shoulder in towards the patient and place your shoulder under the bridge formed by the knee. Bring your hand under the patient's leg and firmly grip the backside or side of the femur.

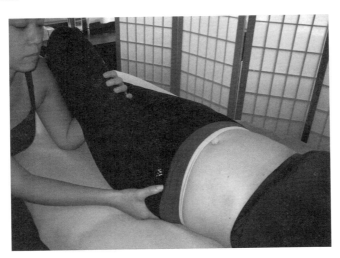

Fig. 14.4   One hand holding the side of the hip, the other holding the leg

I sometimes place the patient's knee up on my shoulder while gripping the leg firmly. This extra support for the patient's leg creates an even stronger illusion that the

112

patient's body is being "fully supported" even though I am only using a very small area of my own body to "control" a fairly large area on the patient.

Now, holding all this area firmly, begin by imperceptibly nudging or *imagining* nudging the ball of the hip farther into the hip socket.

Next, nudge the ball out from the socket.

Then, just as explained with the ball of the shoulder, imagine a clock face, numbered one through twelve, around the hip joint. I usually put the one at the top (towards the person's head) of the socket, and the six down at the bottom (towards the feet) of the socket. On the left side, I put three at the back of the socket, and nine at the front, and fill in the rest of the "clock face" accordingly. On the right side, the three is to the front, etc. Not that it matters.

Notice if there are any areas that do not respond, and give them extra time, or go back to them later, after you've assessed the whole hip area

Hips and sacrum

For the novice, getting a good, supportive grip on the back part of the hip joints, the sacro-iliac joint, can be a bit tricky. Where do you even begin? Happily, there are several techniques for getting the hip joint firmly in control of your hands. The best requires that you be standing up, facing the patient, with the patient lying on his back.

You will start by working on the hip that is farther from you, rather than the closer hip. Reaching for the patient's farther leg, bring the patient's farther knee up while keeping the patient's farther foot flat on the table. And ask the patient to keep it there while you get your hands in place.

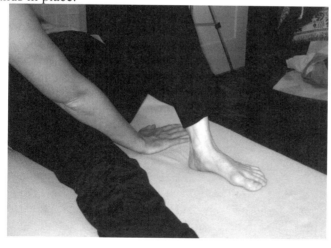

Fig. 14.5   Place your hand under the "bridge" formed by the patient's farther knee

Put your arm – the arm closer to the patient's feet, not the arm closer to the patient's head - under the "bridge" formed by the patient's elevated knee. Place your hand, palm down, on the table on the far side of the bridge.

Place your other arm on the "ASIS" (anterior superior iliac spine): the bit of the hip bone that protrudes out the front in very slender people. Get a firm grip on the ASIS, or maybe reaching around the lateral side of the ASIS, so that you can lift the hip on this side slightly off the table. Gently raise the far hip a mere inch or so off the table

Tell the patient to be limp in the hips – he shouldn't try to "help" the practitioner by lifting the hip high in the air. (If the patient is very large, you may need to ask for his help, but remind him to relax after he's put the hip back down.)

While the hip is raised, slide the other hand, the one that is palm down on the table, under the center of patient's far hip – still palm down, on the table.

Once your hand is centered under the patient's buttock, rotate the "palm down" hand so that your hand is "standing" up: the little-finger side is resting on the table, and the thumb-side is raised up, supporting the patient's hip. This hand position will raise the hip a bit farther in the air. Keep rotating this hand quickly and smoothly until it is fully palm facing up, and then let your upper hand release its lifting hold on the ASIS.

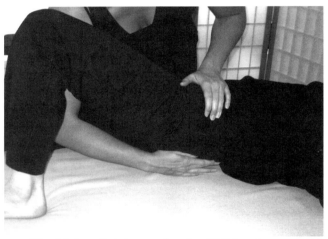

Fig. 14.6   Rotate your hand until it is palm up.

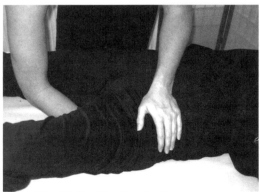

Fig. 14.7   Hand under the sacrum

As the patient's hip drops back down to the table, it will automatically settle down in such a way as to minimize the lumpiness of your lower hand. To do this, the patient's body will automatically center itself over your hand, so that you find yourself with your hand directly under the patient's sacrum. The sacrum is the triangular bone at the base of the spine that joins the two hip bones.

You must practice this move *several* times for it to become smooth and effortless. But once you have mastered it, it is an elegant, quick, and smooth way to position one hand under the sacrum, with no disquieting fumbling in the vicinity of the genitals.

With one hand under the sacrum, you can now place the other hand on the ASIS, which gives you a good starting place to supportively hold while checking on the reflexive movement in the sacro-iliac joint.

Take a moment to imagine the diagonal line of the joint where the far-side of the sacrum meets the far ilium (ilium is singular, ilia is plural. Ili*ac* is the adjective form). I say "far side" because this hand positioning requires that you hold the far hip, rather than the near hip.

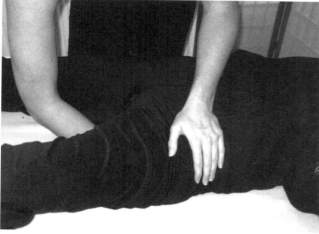

Fig. 14.8 One hand under the sacrum, the other hand on the ASIS, feeling for responsive movement in the sacro-iliac joint

Now you're in position to start nudging, or imagine nudging, that joint.

First, nudge or imagine nudging the joint as if you are compressing the bones more closely together. Remember, these bones meet on a diagonal line. See if there is any response. Imagine you are moving the bones farther apart.

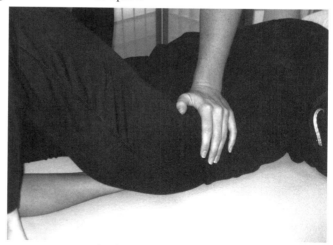

Fig. 14.9 Another view of one hand under the sacrum, the other holding the ASIS

Next, see if the hip bone can move towards the head, relative to the sacrum, which moves towards the feet. Remember, this movement will not be a line that runs parallel to the spine. It is an angled line, so when I say "towards the head" I actually mean "upward, towards the far shoulder." See if there is any response.

Then try moving the ilium in the opposite direction, towards the feet, while the *sacrum* moves towards the head. Again, it is an angled move, not a move that runs parallel to the spine.

Finally, nudge or imagine a nudge that pushes the sacrum ever so slightly forward, towards the front of the body, while nudging the ilium towards the back of the body.

And then the reverse: ilium towards the front, sacrum towards the back.

Remember: all of these moves are extremely subtle. You are not actually moving these bones around. You are merely introducing the slightest of nudges, or even the thought of a movement.

Then, examine/treat the hip on the *opposite* side of the body: stand on the *opposite* side of the table and repeat all the above.

This gentle series of moves can sometimes bring about significant relaxation in the hip joints. If some area does not respond to the gentle suggestions, try making the nudge more gentle, or merely imagining it, or try giving the nudge a tiny *bit* more power – but never enough that the patient can tell what you are doing. If the specific nudge still doesn't garner a response, settle in comfortably for a while and just hold the area, keeping firm pressure from your hands as if they are holding the sacroiliac (SI) joint snugly compressed.

Excellent diagrams of the sacrum, the ilium, and the sacroiliac joint are available online.

Chapter fifteen

The head and spine

The many aspects of head- and spine-holding are worthy of an entire book. In fact, such books have already been written.

If you are going to work on a person's head and spine because you suspect rigidity in those areas or the presence of an unhealed injury, you might do well to buy any of the excellent books already available on the subject of craniosacral therapy.

These books will explain the correct articulations of the skull and spine bones, and suggest the most advantageous placement for the hands.

Of course, these books are just a starting point. Once you get comfortable with your hands on the cranial and spinal bones, you will find that you can branch out on your own, and hold the patient in the places to which your hands are drawn.

You might be able to find a trained craniosacral therapist in your area. But a word of warning: most craniosacral protocols use more force than most dissociated people or people with Parkinson's feel safe with. The books on the subject usually suggest using a very low level of force to pull or push the various cranial and spinal bones, in order to encourage them to relax and drift into the most ideal anatomical positions. While many people truly enjoy this gentle pressure, we have found that many, if not most, of our Parkinson's patients find this "low level pressure" to be far too intrusive.

Therapists trained in this modality have been told that the amount of force they need to use is "minimal" or even "imperceptible." But people who are trying to stay dissociated from the area, and people with Parkinson's with either dissociation or pause mode, will be able to feel these forces and will steel themselves against the intrusion. If your local craniosacral therapist can't use an FSR level of patience and non-directed force, you might be better off just doing this work by yourself.

If you are working from a craniosacral instruction book that instructs you to use light force to push or hold in a given direction, don't. Instead, simply place your hands firmly and supportively in the hand positions recommended in the book, and just sit there. Sometimes a very slight directional pressure *might* be appropriate, but generally, at least for the first few sessions, people with Parkinson's disease find the "gentle" forces suggested in the books to be oppressive, even frightening.

Possibly the best book on the subject is John Upledger's *Craniosacral Therapy*. But be warned, this is a very detailed book, a fairly expensive book, and is oriented towards health professionals. You don't really need all the theory that he uses to validate his ideas about light touch therapy. All you really need to learn is where to place your hands to best provide support. So if you don't want to get into a professional level of craniosacral treatment, I've included the following very quick course in hand positions for craniosacral work.

A very quick course in hand positions for craniosacral work.

The following hand positions are usually the most important ones. Of course, once you get familiar with holding the various parts of someone's head or spine, you will be able to branch out on your own. You will let your hands be your guides as to where to hold and support any places on the head or spine that aren't described below. Well-trained craniosacral therapists work in the same way: they learn the basic holding positions, but as they come to get more comfortable working with cranial bones, they branch out on their own and "do what the patient's body tells them to do."

If you are not familiar with the names of the cranial bones, please research the cranial anatomy by going online for more and better pictures than I could hope to include in this book. I am including photos of the hand positions that can be helpful for holding these areas. Still, for an in-depth understanding of what might move, to where, and why, you might want to read something from the literature that has sprung up around this subject.

Places to hold

1) the occiput
2) the frontal bone
3) the parietal bones
4) the sphenoid bone
5) the sacrum
6) the temporal bones
7) release of diaphragms
8) cervical vertebrae
9) spinal traction

Note: all holding positions assume that the patient is lying down on his back, facing the ceiling.

1. Holding the occiput

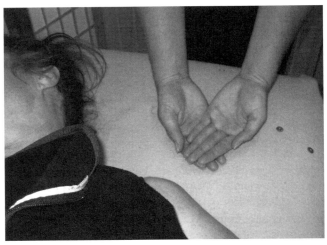

Place your cupped hands under the somewhat spherical "ball" of the occiput. If you're working on a healthy person with no head or neck injuries, you'll probably notice that, if you sit very still, you might feel the occiput rocking towards you and away from you, as it rocks on the top vertebrae in response to the pumping of the sacrum's pumping action. This pumping action moves cerebrospinal fluid. Please practice this on a healthy person.

Fig. 15.1 Showing how the hands will be positioned under the back of the head

People with Parkinson's very often have inhibited flow of cerebrospinal fluid plus rigidity in the neck that can inhibit the pumping motion of the occiput.

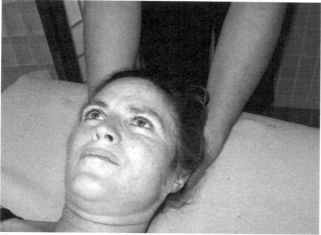

Fig. 15.2 The "cupped" hands seen the in previous photo have been placed under the head, and simply cradle the head. Although this photo shows the therapist standing up, one usually sits while doing this, as you might be holding for a long time before the occiput relaxes and begins gently rocking back and forth.

2. Frontal bone

Place your fourth finger, the "ring" finger, on either side of the frontal bone, in the convenient indentation just superior (closer to the top of the head) to the lateral side of the eyebrows. This bone, if relaxed, might be able to move ever so slightly towards the ceiling. If this bone has sustained an injury, it may have become slightly compacted inwards. An imperceptible movement on your part towards the ceiling might encourage this bone to move to its correct position. Don't *move* the bone around. Hold it. Support it. Maybe do small nudges towards and away from the ceiling. If it *wants* to move, stay with it.

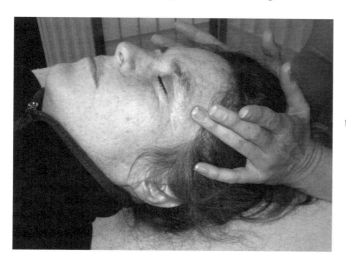

Fig 15.3　Side view of holding the frontal bone with the 4th finger

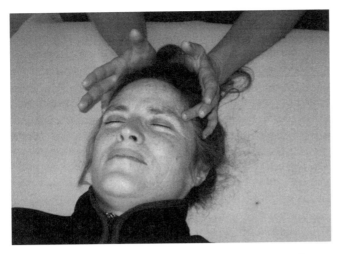

Fig. 15.4   Frontal view of holding the frontal bone with the 4th finger

3. Parietal bones

Place your fingertips where the parietal bones articulate with the temporal bones. The beveled edges of these bones articulate with the temporal bones by sliding under the beveled edge of the temporal bones. A blow to these bones can jam them too far down under the edge of the temporal bones. If this happens, the "too tight" parietal-temporal bone articulations can prevent the temporal bones from rotating freely.

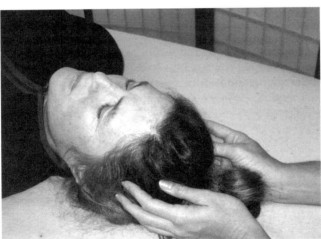

Fig. 15.5   Holding the parietal bone near the suture (joint) with the temporal bone

You may wish to gently *imagine* the parietal bones gently moving towards your own chest as you sit behind the patient's head. This movement will bring the parietals out from under the temporal bones, just a little bit, thus freeing up the temporal bone movements. If these bones feel stuck, maybe nudge them further under, or away from, the temporal bones. You are not trying to move the bones, per se, but to encourage them to relax and thus be able to move back into their best position.

4. Sphenoid

Rest your thumbs on the sides of the face, just posterior to the eyes, in the small indentation in the skull.

DO NOT nudge these bones in any direction. If you displace the sphenoid bone in the slightest, the person may get a headache, poor visual focus, and other problems. So just rest your thumbs in this spot.

If the sphenoid bone wants to move of its own accord, allow it to do so. In many cases of sphenoid displacement, the bone has moved too far posteriorly (towards the back of the head), and will want to move anteriorly, towards the front of the face. But sometimes it needs to move side to side, or one side up and the other side down, or posteriorly.

When I teach craniosacral protocal, the move most likely to lead to head problems and complaints on the following day is pushing or shoving on the sphenoid. Use no force on the sphenoid area. Perfect balance in this area is crucial. Be careful with this one.

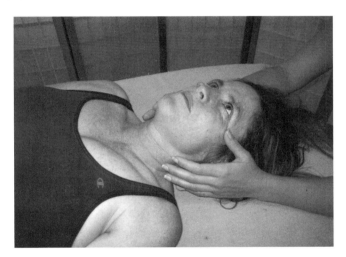

Fig. 15.6   Thumbs resting on the sphenoid bone. In this photo, it almost appears as if the thumbs are pushing towards the jaw – they are not. The thumbs are just sitting, not pushing in any direction.

As the sphenoid bone relaxes, it will usually move anteriorly (towards the ceiling, in the above photo.

5. Sacrum

To hold the sacrum, use the same technique described in the previous chapter for getting your hands in the right position to work on the sacroiliac joint. Once you have got your "under" hand positioned nicely under the patient's sacrum, place your upper hand on the patient's abdomen, as close to the pubic bone as you and the patient feel comfortable with. Rest a bit with your hands in this position, and maybe nudge your hands closer together a few times. Support in this position can sometimes allow muscles in the pelvic floor to relax, which then allows the sacrum to position itself more correctly.

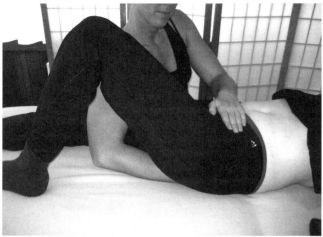

Fig. 15.7   One hand under the sacrum, the upper hand on the abdomen, approaching the pubic bone

6. Temporal bones

Place your fingers in a "circle" around the "ear bone" (the bone that underlies the ear) – not on the ear itself. Your fingers will need to be "under" the ear, or you might say, resting on the skin of the skull, so that you can get your fingers as close to the center of the temporal bone as possible.

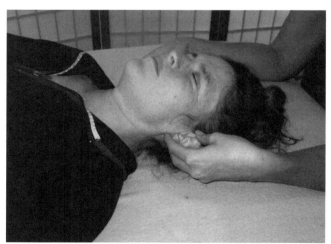

Fig. 15.8   Fingers on the temporal bone: the skin under the ear

With your hands in this position, you might be able to every so slightly rotate the skin over the temporal bones around the axis of the ear hole. If you imagine the somewhat

122

round temporal bone as being the face of the clock, you should be able to move the skin over the temporal bones ever-so-slightly clockwise and counterclockwise. Never use force – if the skin over the ears doesn't want to rotate, then just imagine a rotation.

The temporal bones evolved from our gills. Like gills, they move in a pumping motion, with every breath.

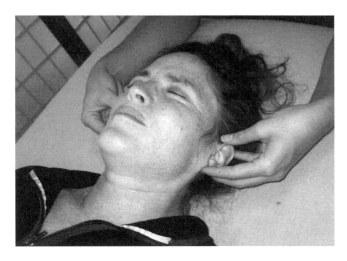

Fig. 15.9   Another view of holding the temporals

In a healthy person with no excessive muscle tensions in the head or spine, the temporal bones rotate slightly backwards with every exhalation, and forward with every inhalation. In this case, "backwards" means "the right ear moves counter-clockwise if you are standing on the patient's right side, looking at the right ear, and the reverse, on the left.

Another way of thinking of it is that top ("superior," closer to the top of the head) part of the temporal bones moves towards the back of the head with each exhalation while the bottom of the temporal bone moves towards the chin.

This bone often gets stuck via muscle spasm if a person has a spasm in the psoas muscle, in the back. Even a slight psoas muscle spasm will pull the spine to the side. In order to keep one's eyes level with the ground, a deep, subconscious instinct, a person with spasm in the psoas muscle will very often, without realizing it, choose to use a spasm of the opposite-side temporal bone muscles to make the eyes stay level. This can cause mild headache and is also the number one cause of ear ringing.[1]

---

[1] If you have a patient with recent-onset ear-ringing, you can usually get rid of it in one or two sessions by first getting rid of the psoas muscle spasm, and then teaching the patient how to manually rotate his temporal bones in time with his exhalations. Have the patient place his hands on his own temporal bones and gently rotate them backwards while exhaling. He should do this three times in a row, several times a day. If the ear ringing has been going on for weeks, months, or years, it may take several weeks or months for the patient's body to completely unlearn the habit of spasm in the temporal bone. Also, the patient's psoas spasm *must* be released. The psoas-spasm release technique is discussed in the next chapter.

7. Diaphragms

Two muscular "diaphragms" might be holding tension: one is under the lungs, the other is the group of muscles at the top of the lungs, at the bottom of the throat.

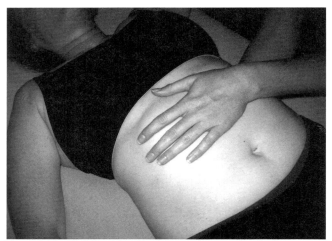

Fig. 15.10   Holding the diaphragm that works the lungs

To release tension in the diaphragm below the lungs, place one hand on the front of the torso, just below the sternum (Fig. 15.10) and the other hand under the spine, directly beneath the upper hand. Hold for a bit, and maybe nudge the hands together for a split second, to see if the muscles between your hands can relax. As always, if there is movement, keep your hands in good contact and follow the movement with your hands, maintaining the support.

The next "diaphragm," or collection of muscles that makes a circle, is around the top of the rib cage: the thoracic inlet. Place one hand on the top of the sternum and the other hand underneath the first hand.

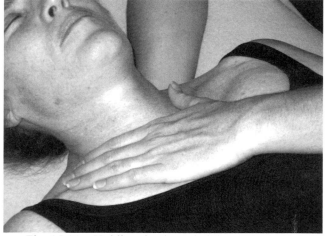

Fig. 15.11   Holding the thoracic inlet

8. Cervical vertebrae

Place your hands gently on either side of the patient's neck, and just hold. Do not try to move or "adjust" anything! The alignments of these bones are very precise. You can do real harm by interfering with these bones. This is a book for do-it-yourselfers, as well as medical students. Unless you are medically licensed to move these bones, do not do so. However, just placing your hands on either side of the neck can very often give enough support so that the neck bones, if slightly out of place or the muscles, if slightly in spasm, will move and relax back into their correct places.

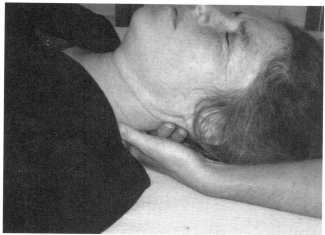

Fig. 15.12   Holding the neck (cervical vertebrae)

9. Spinal traction

Placing one hand under the patient's sacrum, as shown earlier, very, very, very gently *imagine* that you are pulling the sacrum towards the feet. You can imagine that the spine is loosening at each vertebra. You can even count the five lumbar, twelve thoracic, and seven neck vertebrae as you imagine that each one, in turn, is gently moving towards the feet, creating a tiny distance between each vertebrae, one at a time. Even if you only *imagine* that you are pulling the sacrum towards the feet, the patient may feel a genuine lengthening of the spine, and often feel a bit taller after this treatment.

On the other hand, if you actually *pull* on the patient's spine, he may well tighten up in his spine, to resist you.

Next, while sitting at the head of the table on which the patient is lying, so that you are behind the patient's head, with the top of the patient's head facing you, place your hands on either side of the patient's head, and imagine, *imagine,* that you are pulling the head oh-so-slighly off of the topmost vertebra by pulling the patient's head towards your chest. Then, continue to imagine the stretch continuing down the patient's spine, going past the seven cervicals, the twelve thoracics, and the five lumbar vertebrae, until your reach the sacrum.

At this point, if your focus has migrated, with your imagination, all the way down to the sacrum, you might be even able to feel the gentle back and forth movement in the sacrum, as it pumps the cerebrospinal fluid.

In all of the above holding positions, place your hands on the patient gently, and remove your hands gently. If the patient's body seems to be magnetically pulling on your hands, then sit with your hands in that position until the patient "lets go" of you, and then gently, respectfully, remove your hands.

It's OK to go to a professional

The above information is not meant to imply that anyone can and should feel comfortable performing craniosacral therapy on friends and loved ones. The above information has been provided because some Parkinson's patients have head, spine, and neck injuries *and* they do not live anywhere near a professional craniosacral therapist. For these people, the above, introductory, modified craniosacral therapy holding positions have been provided.

If you live in an area where craniosacral therapists are easy to find on the internet, I highly recommend you use their services.

However, if you are working with a Parkinson's patient, you must let the therapist know right from the beginning that your PD patient finds the "extremely light pressure" that is "standard" is going to be far too intrusive. Ask the practitioner to just place his hands in the usual positions for the standard protocol and keep them there for a while, in each of the positions, holding firmly, and noticing if the bones spontaneously do any moving on their own.

If the bones do move, great. But if there are areas that, to the experienced hands of the craniosacral therapist, feel "stuck," ask him to either just sit there at those positions, not moving, or else show you which hand positions elicited no response, or a "stuck" response.

Then, you can go home and practice holding these particular areas for an hour at a stretch, which may be what your patient actually needs in order to release in these areas.

If your craniosacral therapist responds to your request by saying, "I don't need to modify my technique: I only use a little pressure to help things move around. It won't be a problem," then ask for a referral to a different craniosacral therapist. Or let the cransiosacral therapist do a few sessions on the patient while you take notes regarding the hand positions – and then go home and practice those hand positions with *no* overt moving of the craniosacral bones – and see which form of treatment your patient prefers.

I've had Parkinson's patients who have seen craniosacral therapists who used "minimal pressure" or "only five grams of pressure." Some of these patients have felt so threatened by that "minimal pressure" that they could feel themselves locking down *more* rigidly or defensively than normal in order to deal with the impositions of the craniosacral therapist. The people with Parkinson's who feel this way just can't help it: their strong desire to not be "messed with" is stronger than their desire to relax.

If the craniosacral therapist cannot understand this, then find someone else.

As an aside, I very strongly recommend that all my Yin Tui Na students at the acupuncture college take a professional craniosacral class. After taking a weekend craniosacral class, my Yin Tui Na students who've already spent a few months working on a few Parkinson's patients invariably report back to me saying things like, "The other students in the craniosacral class were really having a hard time feeling the subtle rhythms and cerebrospinal fluid movements, they kept asking what it was they were looking for. They were having a really hard time feeling *anything*. But it was so *easy* for all of us who've had the FSR class. Heck, those cerebrospinal movements were overt, *glaring*, compared to the tiny movements, or the utter non-responsiveness, of our Parkinson's patients!"

My students, by working with Parkinson's patient via sitting for an hour at a time feeling next-to-nothing, by patiently supporting these patients with practically rigid bodies, had become so much more "tuned in" to subtle changes and rhythms that the so-called "subtle" and "barely discernable" movements of basic craniosacral therapy were, to them, obvious or even glaring. And the amounts of pressure that they were instructed to use in these classes seemed to my students to be almost offensive.

They felt that the supportive, un-intrusive holding that they had been learning in their FSR classes was far more likely to trigger the release of a stuck holding pattern than the so-called "gentle" or "minimal" amounts of pressure advocated by their craniosacral teachers.

Since I took my first craniosacral class back in the early 1990s, gentler forms of craniosacral therapy have been "invented." There are now several schools of craniosacral therapy that teach the extremely non-invasive, nothin' but holding methods that we use in FSR. Still, it seems that the majority of craniosacral therapists study the "gentle pressure" methods – which is far too much intrusion for many people with dissociated injuries or for people with Parkinson's.

Most practitioners of manual therapy, looking over the extensive scale of body work, ranging from vigorous and manipulative all the way to subtle and gentle, consider craniosacral work to be at the extreme far end of subtle.

But FSR, which very often ends up consisting of firmly holding while apparently doing "nothing at all" is even more subtle. And sometimes, doing "nothing at all" is the only way to unlock the fear and dissociation that has kept a traumatized body part shut down for decades.

Massage therapists

On paper, FSR sounds easy: hold firmly and don't do anything, and don't impose your thoughts on the patient. But it can be very, very difficult to do this.

Curiously, in my experience, some of the people who've had the hardest time mastering FSR have been professional massage therapists. Within a few minutes of supportively holding, they want to get busy "doing something."

Several of them have complained to me with something along the lines of, "How can I justify getting payment for not *doing* anything?"

I point out to them that, by firmly holding and remaining motionless for long periods of time, they are providing a very rare and skilled service. This is a service that many people with unhealed injury desperately need. But the people trained primarily in gross massage techniques are dubious that they can ask for money for "doing nothing."

They have been trained to push and shove. And unless they are allowed to push and shove, some massage therapists, though certainly not all, feel that they aren't doing anything worthwhile.

If you are feeling awkward about "doing nothing" while doing Yin Tui Na, please keep in mind that you are doing something that requires patience and confidence. You are not "doing nothing." And if it comes to that, as one of my colleagues pointed out, "Some people "do nothing" better than others."

So if you are in need of Yin Tui Na type therapies and are planning to look for a health professional who will learn FSR or other forms of Yin Tui Na on your behalf, do not *assume* that just any massage therapist will be your best bet.

On the other hand, some excellent FSR therapists have come from the ranks of massage therapists who *do* understand the power of supportive, non-invasive contact.

And then again, ultimately, supportive holding of an injured person is one of the most basic of human instincts. Almost all of us know to hold an injured or frightened infant or young child closely, in a snug embrace. And most of us know how to tell when the infant or child no longer needs to be held.

You do *not* need to be a health professional to learn these techniques and quickly master them. You just need to be willing to go slowly and patiently, without getting emotionally involved in "how fast" the patient is going to heal, or whether or not you are "doing it" correctly. After all, if you are "doing" anything, you are very likely doing too much. Hold the patient firmly, and let him come, in his own time, to his own conclusions about whether or not he feels safe enough to start paying attention to, and *feeling*, and *recovering* from his injury, pain, and fear.

Chapter sixteen

Psoas muscle release

A spasm in the psoas (pronounced SO-as) muscle is a very, very common occurrence. The majority of back pain problems and sacroiliac problems have their origin in psoas muscle spasm.

The psoas is one of the longest muscles in the body. At its top end, it attaches to the spine up by the lung's diaphragm, and connects, at the lower end, at the top of the femur, the large bone of the upper leg.

The ideal use of this muscle is raising the thigh. Tightening this muscle is said to "decrease the angle of the upper leg and torso."

For example, if you are standing up straight, the "angle" of the torso junction with the thigh is 180°. When your thigh is raised, such as when you are sitting, the angle is decreased to approximately 90°.

Hurting your back

The problem in humans is that they tend to use the psoas muscle to bend forward. This motion also decreases the angle between the torso and thigh: the job of the psoas muscle. However, this muscle was never designed to lever the whole mass of the torso and head. In quadrupeds, this muscle is designed to lift the leg: in a quadruped, the leg is a small percentage of the overall body.

In humans, we might bend forward by tightening the psoas, but the torso and head is a *large* percentage of the overall body in a human. The psoas muscle can over-react to the job, tighten up too much, and then go into spasm – from which it doesn't automatically release. If we are leaning even a bit to one side or the other, one side's psoas muscle will tighten more than the other side – and might go into spasm, pulling the back violently to one side. When it does this, the nerves that emerge from between the vertebrae can get painfully squeezed: "back pain."

Sometimes, the sacrum even gets pulled to one side by the power of the psoas muscle. In these cases, the nerves in the sacrum can get squeezed (overstimulated), causing a pain sensation that might seem to originate anywhere from the hip to the toe. But even if the pain sensation seems to be coming from the hip, knee, or toe, the actual location of the problem is usually in the sacroiliac joint, which can be tweaked by a spastic psoas muscle. If the psoas muscle can be made to relax, the vertebrae can go back to their correct positions. The pain signals being created by squeezed nerves, signals that incorrectly suggest that the problem is in the toes, the mid back, or even up by the lungs, will cease.

So many people say, "I just bent down to pick up a paper clip, and my back went out!" The problem is not the weight that was lifted, but the quick, thoughtless, assymetrical manner in which the person bent down in the first place.

It is much better to lower the torso towards the ground by bending at the knees, or by very carefully, mindfully, bending equally with both left and right sides, tightening the psoas to lower the torso and then, carefully, gently, symmetrically loosening it again as we stand back up.

Diagnosing a psoas spasm

If you suspect a psoas spasm, do this easy diagnostic test. Lie flat on your back with the knees bent, feet flat on the floor. Let the knees flop laterally, to the outer sides. The left knee flops to the left, the right knee flops to the right. If one or both legs do not flop easily, there is probably some amount of psoas spasm on the side of the body that fails to flop. If, while relaxing on your back, your knees stay tightly together, there's almost always a psoas spasm holding those knees in place. When the psoas muscle is relaxed, the hip/leg joint is relaxed and opens wide. The tighter the psoas is, the more the knee(s) will be pulled close to the midline.

Treating a psoas spasm

To treat a psoas spasm, first make sure the patient's spine is as straight as possible. (See "spinal traction," in the previous chapter, p. 123.) Then, have the patient, who is lying down, bend one knee, with his foot flat on the table.

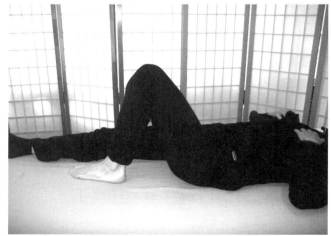

Fig. 16.1   Knee bent, foot flat on the table

The patient *or* the health practitioner should gently press down with his fingers at the psoas release point: midway between his belly-button and the superior (closer to the head) end of the ASIS (the front part of the hip bone that sticks out in front on slender people.

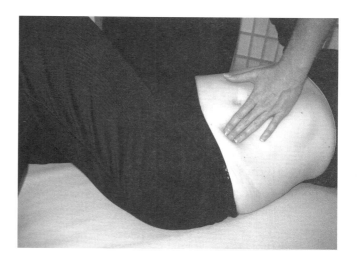

Fig. 16.2 Psoas-release point: mid-way between the belly button and the upper end of the ASIS

While massaging the psoas release point on his abdomen, the patient or practitioner must simultaneously move the patient's bent knee towards the midline of his body. The "midline" is an imaginary line that travels from the nose, down past the belly-button, ending between the feet. This imaginary line divides the body into left side and right side.

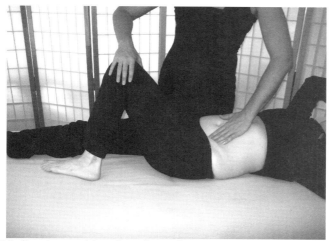

Fig. 16.3 Starting position: knee bent, fingers massaging the psoas-spasm point.

Again: the patient or the practitioner brings the bent knee gently towards the midline and gently back to its original upright position, all the while massaging the psoas release point on the abdomen.

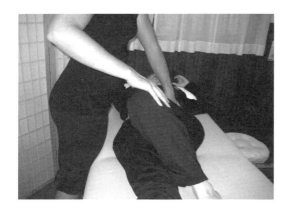 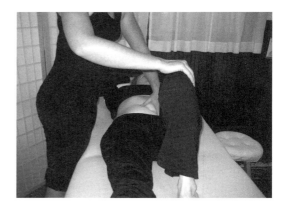

Fig.s 16.4 and 16.5   Bringing the knee to the midline and then returning it to upright, while massaging the psoas-release point

Repeat the "knee-to-midline and then back to upright" movement ten times, massaging the psoas-release point the whole time. You should spend about one second on each of the midline-to-upright moves.

After doing this ten times, *then* you may test your treatment by *gently* moving the bent knee out towards the side (laterally). Do *not* force the knee out to the lateral side. It should move laterally more easily than before. If a psoas spasm is very tight, it may still be difficult for the patient to move the bent knee laterally, but it might be easier than before. After doing the above psoas relaxation technique, the patient may suddenly find it *far* easier to move the knee laterally than it has been in a long, long time. However, if the knee is still unable to move laterally easily, without forcing it, then *repeat* the above.

With a few patients with very tight psoas spasms, I've had to repeat this release sequence for half an hour before the muscles have started to relax.

I had a fourteen-year old patient with severe chronic back pain. When her psoas muscle finally relaxed, after nearly an hour of my bringing her bent knees back and forth, while massaging the abdominal "psoas release" point, she was astonished.

She told her mother and me, "I didn't know people could move their knees and legs *outward*!"

Psoas release part two: releasing the compensation mechanism

As mentioned in the previous chapter, a person with a psoas spasm will usually have a compensating spasm somewhere else in his body – a compensation designed to enable the eyes to be horizontal with the ground in spite of the slight spinal contortion from the psoas spasm. Our bodies will do just about anything to keep the eyes horizontal to the ground.

This compensating spasm is typically in the temporal bones, though it can sometimes be found in the shoulder, neck, or upper torso.

After the psoas muscle has been relaxed, then you can oh-so-gently rotate the temporal bones to get them to stop being in spasm. After performing the psoas release *and* temporal release on the patient, teach the patient how to do this to himself. He should do both the psoas and temporal releases at least twice a day. Since he needs to lie down to do these, suggest that he do them when he's already lying down: before he gets out of bed in the morning and when he goes to bed at night.

This little "trick" can be enormously helpful. So many people have aches and pains in their back, side, head, neck, or while taking a deep breath, and so on, pains that are being caused by a psoas muscle spasm.

If the spasm quickly resumes after the patient stands up from the treatment table, then you have one of two situations going on: either the compensating spasm was not located in the temporal bones, and you will need to track it down by holding, with FSR, the shoulders, neck, and upper torso. Or, the vertebrae are out of alignment, forcing the psoas back into spasm. If this seems to be the case, and it may well be, with severe spasms, you may want to redo the psoas sequence a few times and then traction the spine a few times, as taught in the previous chapter. After tractioning, perform the psoas release again a few times.

This gentle but powerful exercise is one of the most important tools in my acupuncturist's toolbox. I find myself teaching this exercise to patients several times a week. If they are dutiful about practicing it twice a day, their back problems will quickly resolve and not return, even if they have a long history of their backs "going out."

Prevent it from happening in the future

Your patients will also benefit enormously from learning to tighten their lumbar quadratis muscles for a minute or two, several times a day. These muscles are tightened when a person sits on the floor with his knees out to the sides, as when doing the yoga asana called "lotus position."

The psoas muscles and the lumbar quadratis muscles are an oppositional pair: when one relaxes, the other tightens, and vice versa.

When a person sits in chairs, or cars, or in other postures that keep the knees somewhat close together while the thighs are at a ninety-degree angle to the torso, his psoas muscles are tight and his lumbar quadratis muscles are therefore relaxed.

A healthy person *should* spend most of his sitting time with his knees as far apart as possible: with his lumbar quadratis tightened and his psoas relaxed - just the opposite of how westerners sit.

If a person can train himself to be aware of his lumbar quadratis muscles, and tighten them for a few seconds, a few times every day, or every ten minutes while driving in the car, he will *not* develop the classic westerner's back pain. He will be able to easily get out of a car and stand straight up even after driving for hours, even if he used to have a history of back spasm or if he's "elderly" (whatever that means).

I describe the tightening of the lumbar quads to patients by saying, "It's the muscle on your backside that attaches the top / back of your hip bones to your lowest ribs. If you move like you are trying to bring the top / back of your hip bones up to your ribs, your back will arch a bit, as if you are starting to do a back bend. Your stomach will stick out in front, just a bit.

The lumbar quads are also the muscles that tighten when you arch your back while swimming the breast stroke.

As you tighten these left and right side muscles the first few times, there will be a gently sore sensation at the top of your hip bones. The pulling sensation is here, at the top / back of your hips bones. You should *not* feel the pull at the opposite end of the muscle, on your ribs.

Chapter seventeen

Fun facts about YinTui Na

These next few chapters might seem a bit extraneous. Or introductory. They might just as well have been placed near the front of the book as here, near the end.

I decided to place this non-crucial information here at the back to allow readers to more quickly cut to the chase and get started on actually practicing Tui Na. But having starting practicing, you might now have some questions. These chapters answer the most frequently asked questions.

The disappearance of Yin Tui Na

You might have wondered why you can't find anyone in your area that does Yin Tui Na. Chinese politics of the mid-twentieth century has a lot to do with that.

More than twenty years ago, after having gotten my Master's degree in Chinese medicine, I was re-visiting my old school's library when I came across a book titled *Tui Na: Chinese Massage*. The book's intro claimed that the text was a direct translation of the text approved for use in one of the top Chinese Medical schools. (The poor quality of the translation – a characteristic of all the recently translated texts, at that time – made a convincing case for this claim.)

The book started by stating that Tui Na is an ancient art, preceding the development of acupuncture: "The unearthed oracle inscriptions …of the Shang dynasty record that the female witch doctor, Bi, could treat patients with massage [Tui Na]."[1]

The introduction of the book then proudly explained that both Yin and Yang forms of Tui Na were a part of the rich cultural heritage of China. It explained further that Yang techniques were overt, and were usually used when an injury was new and painful: "bright, or "Yang." Yin techniques were subtle. They were more likely to be used if an injury was old, forgotten, and painless. "Old," "dark," and "hidden" are all "Yin" qualities.

The introduction went on and on for several pages with generalities about the difference between Yin and Yang types of Tui Na, together with repeated assurances that all known techniques, ranging from very Yin to very Yang, were presented in the book.

However, when I flipped through the book, I discovered that the introduction was incorrect. The book contained only *very* Yang techniques: overt "cracking" or twisting of the spine to relieve back pain, violent snapping motions of the neck for displaced cervical vertebrae, and so on.

---

[1] *Chinese Massage*; Publishing House of Shanghai College of Traditional Chinese Medicine; Shanghai; 1988; p.2.

Note: the Shang dynasty dates from approximately 1766 BC to 1027 BC. The actual text would have said that Bi could treat patients with *Tui Na*. Again, the use of the word "massage" when translating into the English is *not* accurate.

There was no mention *anywhere* in the book about gentler techniques such as skin-rolling, acupressure, or the deeply supportive, gentle type of holding that can bring together and reset, perfectly, painlessly, the ends of a broken bone, or the firm support that can bring the patient's attention, and therefore healing, to an injury that had been long ignored.

I pored through that book, looking for *any* Yin techniques, based on the description in the introduction. I inquired in the school's library and even the main office as to whether the Yin techniques might be in a separate volume. No, there was no missing volume. This was a translation of the entire book, the latest official version of Chinese government-approved medical Tui Na.

I learned, a few years later, that *Yin* Tui Na had been intentionally dropped from the Officially Approved Texts. This disappearance probably occurred because, at some point in the mid-twentieth century, the light touch therapies were deemed "not scientific enough," and even "too charismatic" (related more to the practitioner's charm than any medical science). At any rate, by government decree, Yin Tui Na was no longer taught. Officially, it no longer *existed*.

Yin Tui Na had been left in the *introduction* to the texts, most likely by accident.

This disappearance probably occurred around the same time that channel theory, the basis of all Chinese medicine, was made illegal, in the mid-twentieth century. The Chinese government has long been extremely sensitive to mockery of its medicine from western doctors. Acupuncture itself has been made illegal three times in the last hundred and fifty years. I am not at all surprised that Yin Tui Na, which can appear to bring about spontaneous, "inexplicable" healing responses, was dropped from the books and, according to Chinese colleagues, made *illegal*.

Stumbling across Yin Tui Na

My own medical practice just happened to develop in a direction that required the application of *very* Yin Tui Na – although I had no idea that the techniques I was doing had a traditional Chinese *name*. I was working with patients with Parkinson's disease, many of whom had dissociated or were on pause from injuries or traumas.

As mentioned earlier, many of these patients had injuries that, in many cases, had never hurt – or had "never happened" – usually because they had occurred during a traumatic situation and the injury, being the lesser of two traumas, was never addressed.

Very often, patients did not want these injuries touched by me, or by anyone. Many patients, terrified at the idea of therapy in the injured area, said things like, "No one has ever touched my left foot." Or, "I never even let my spouse *look* at my foot."

Although I did not realize at the time that I myself was manifesting a few dozen early-stage symptoms of Parkinson's, I was strangely sympathetic to people not wanting to be touched or "messed with." I felt the same way. *Very* strongly.

And yet, in order for me to gently draw the patient's attention to their obviously (obvious to *me*) unhealed injuries, thus ending decades of dissociation and electrical currents running the wrong way under the skin, I found myself using extremely Yin Tui Na: nothing but very firm, utter support. I placed my hands on either side of the injured area and simply held it for an hour at a stretch, once a week, until the displaced tissues began to move of their own accord under my hands, or until the patient suddenly exclaimed something like "Ouch! My ankle feels smashed!"

Years earlier, when I was getting my Master's degree in Chinese medicine, my shiatsu (Japanese "massage" that focuses on acupoints) professor had demonstrated a variation of shiatsu that consisted of simple holding. He referred to this technique as "Support." He didn't provide an official Asian name for his technique.

A year or two after graduating, I discovered, in the introduction of the book *Tui Na: Chinese Massage,* that *Yin* Tui Na was the Traditional Chinese Medicine name for work on "old, painless, forgotten injuries," the kind of injuries that I was seeing in my Parkinson's patients.

At the same time, the techniques I *instinctively* was using to treat the injuries of my Parkinson's patients had been based, in part, on the "support technique" I'd learned in the Shiatsu class and was also based in part on the way *I* would want to be therapeutically *manipulated*: not at all.

However, as mentioned previously, although a general description of these types of techniques was in the *introduction* to the official book of Chinese Tui Na, including *when* to use *which* types of techniques, the actual techniques themselves had disappeared from the *modern* Chinese medicine cannon. I had *no* idea what these Yin-type techniques might look like.

The *Yin* techniques were no longer being taught in *Chinese* schools of Tui Na. As I later learned, they had ceased to exist. In China, they were illegal.

But my school's *Japanese* teacher of hands-on therapeutic shiatsu techniques had also taught us about non-manipulative *support* with the hands, as opposed to *manipulating* with the hands. He had no special name for the supportive holding that he did, but his results were legendary.

I never suspected that the illegal techniques of "Yi Tui Na" and the various types of "supportive holding" techniques of my teacher were actually one and the same.

Choosing a name for a technique

In 1998, when I first wrote up an article about the results I was getting in treating the "painless, often forgotten" injuries of my Parkinson's patients, my article briefly described the hands-on "support" technique I was using.[1]

---

[1] I have come across many doctors and health practitioners who do not believe that any person can have an injury and not feel the pain of it. However, neurologists have *long* recognized that certain injuries, inherently life-threatening, do *not* manifest pain, at first. Spinal cord injuries, removal of a limb, and stroke are three types of injury that might *not* hurt for the first few days, and usually, for much longer than that.

In the case of spinal cord injuries, approximately 75% of patients begin to feel the delayed pain between 72 hours and one *year*. The remaining 25% might feel the pain sometime between one year and several decades following the injury – or never.

Years after a spinal cord injury, long after all movement function has been restored, a person may suddenly experience the classic pain of spinal cord injury: terrible pressure in the head, ripping pains in the neck and shoulders, searing pain in the hips or legs (depending on where the spinal cord was injured) – and may have no way of knowing that this is pain that was experienced during the injury and put "on hold" in the brain until such time as the person had the leisure and safety to deal with it.

The editor of the journal I was aiming for was brilliant, detail-obsessed, and gloriously nit-picking. The *American Journal of Acupuncture* is now defunct, but at that time, it was the most respected, longest-running (twenty-five years) *English* language peer-reviewed journal of Chinese Medicine in the world. The editor told me that the hands-on technique I was describing was a "Yin" type of Tui Na.

I'd had no idea. After all, the only book I'd ever seen that even mentioned the words "Yin Tui Na," in the intro, had included *no* information about Yin techniques in the text.

Still, the book had said that Yin Tui Na was used when injuries were old, painless, and even forgotten. That fit my patients to a T.

I accepted the editor's assertion, and from that point on, in my medical practice, I referred to this work, and any light-touch variations such as craniosacral therapy, as Yin Tui Na. Happily, this gave me the convenience of keeping all my hands-on treatment modalities under the Chinese medicine term "Tui Na." This also kept all my treatments under the umbrella of the legal "scope of practice" of an acupuncturist. In California, at any rate, an acupuncturist's scope of practice includes Tui Na.

I was happily surprised to see how my patients responded to this new label for the work that I'd been performing on with them. Prior to labeling the holding technique "Yin Tui Na," I had been merely holding their injuries in some very slow, boring, albeit effective, fashion.

Because I am an acupuncturist, my patients had often asked me how my holding technique was related to traditional Chinese medicine. I had no answer.

After learning from my new editor, I could casually mention that the technique being used was "a Yin form of Tui Na." My patients *loved* it.

They could even search for "Tui Na" on their computers and find articles, so they knew I wasn't just making things up. I no longer underestimate the power of an "official" name.

In 2008, ten years after my first article was published in the *American Journal of Acupuncture*, after I'd published books describing Yin Tui Na techniques and had lectured on the subject in the USA and abroad, I was thrilled to learn, from an acupuncturist attending one of my lectures, that people in China were, once again, *openly* using Yin Tui Na techniques. I cannot verify this student's report, but he said that, for many long years, the subtle Yin forms of hands-on healing work had been banned from the official medical protcols...but health practitioners had continued to perform it in secret. Now, at the beginning of the new millennium, I learned that Yin Tui Na was, once again, being practiced openly as a medical procedure.

In the case of stroke, the pressure in the brain actually causes pain, but this pain is "put on hold" in the brain and does not register, in many cases. However, some people do experience the pain of pressure in the head many months or years after having a stroke. The pain at the severance site of a removed limb may not occur for several weeks or several years after the removal of a limb. (This is different from the phantom limb experience in which people register sensations from the missing limb.)

In my own acupuncture practice, I find that unhealed, long-forgotten, even "painless" injuries, together with mental stances such as dissociation and pause are very common reasons for the body to be unable to heal itself, and are *very* often at the root of movement disorders and chronic pain situations.

Evidently, by the early twenty-*first* century, as the Chinese government officials basked in the burgeoning international support for acupuncture, Qi Gong, and other esoteric practices that had all been banned in China at one time or another (because they invited mockery from the more "scientific" western countries), even subtle medical techniques such as Yin Tui Na were once again out in the open.

I do not know if Yin Tui Na techniques have regained their rightful place in the Chinese medical schools and text books. I do hope that the written material regarding Yin Tui Na was only locked up, and not destroyed. At any rate, we westerners can now state with assurance and confidence that hands-on healing techniques at the more subtle, less intrusive, less-directed (Yin) end of the spectrum are in fact techniques of Chinese medicine, just as much as the bone-snapping, body-jerking (Yang) forms. For acupuncturists, in many states and countries, these gentle forms of support are allowable according to our scope-of-practice laws: laws that permit us to perform "Tui Na," but which never specify what *types* of Tui Na.

What's in a name?

When I started working on the very first edition of this book, I asked the Chinese doctors and teachers at my California acupuncture college for their definitions of Tui Na. My teachers were all practicing acupuncturists. One teacher, an MD in pediatrics from Shanghai, said, "Tui Na means Pediatric Finger Massage: skin rolling." An MD/ Ph.D. in Chinese medicine from Guandong (Canton) said, "It means all forms of Chinese massage." An MD from elsewhere in southern China said, "It cannot be translated. Tui Na means Tui Na." An MD from Shanghai said, "It means bone medicine." Another MD from Shanghai said, "It means bone massage."

My friend Sue, who was an accountant in southern China and now owns a Chinese restaurant in California, gave this non-medical translation: "Tui Na is a doing word, it is a word that means you do something, and then there is a result. It means moving, doing, and then it brings something out that wasn't there before. So then you have something. Because you did something, this way." She moved her hands in a slow, open and shut, back and forth pattern to demonstrate.

Back in the 1980s, when I started working on a Master's degree in Chinese medicine, the most common classroom definitions of Tui Na were "bone medicine" or "skin rolling/pediatric massage." The latter is a relatively new meaning of Tui Na, going back only to the Yuan dynasty. During the Yuan period (1271-1368), the Tui Na/massage department of medicine came under the administration of the bone-setting department. A department of pediatrics was opened also and incorporated into the Tui Na department, making "skin rolling techniques" an official part of the government-approved Chinese medical protocols.[1]

Today, as mentioned in the opening chapter, Tui Na is the name given to almost any form of physical-touch work in which the doctor makes intentional hand contact with

---

[1] *Chinese Massage*; Publishing House of Shanghai College of Traditional Chinese Medicine; Shanghai; 1988; p.12.

the patient. Technically, even acupressure, a process in which acupoints are stimulated by finger pressure, should be considered a form of Tui Na.

As for the bone-setting applications of Yin Tui Na, it is almost never used in western countries. In western countries, the re-setting of broken bones is nearly always done in a western medical clinic or a hospital's emergency room.

But maybe in the future…?

Chapter eighteen

Studying with the masters

When I was getting my master's degree in Traditional Chinese medicine, students were required to take two classes in Tui Na and/or Asian-style massage.

I was so fortunate as to have classes with one of the most brilliant "massage" therapists in, I think, the world. I put the word massage in quotes because the class that Shinzo Fujimaki Sensei was teaching was officially titled "Shiatsu Massage." However, what he taught us was nothing like the usual acupressure poking and prodding that is normally associated with Shiatsu.

Master Fujimaki was so in demand for his "massage" therapy that his appointment calendar was always booked at least three months in advance. His clients testified that his treatments had removed problems ranging from chronic pain to cancerous tumors, asthma, and a long list of other "incurable" ailments.

As a teacher, he worked very hard to convey to us the *essence* of what he was doing and *why*. Many of my fellow students did *not* like his class. Their complaint usually ran something like: "He is wasting our time telling us about his ideas. I don't get it. I just want to learn which place to push on to cure which problems. Fujimaki never tells us anything *practical*."

But many other students, myself included, considered our classes with Master Fujimaki to be some of the most important foundation-stone hours of our entire school career.

Shinzo Fujimaki was a supple and powerful early-middle-aged man with an always radiant smile. He was also an aikido master. When I saw him, now and then, striding along the cliff top walk-ways of our ocean-side city, his stride evoked images of tigers and horses, as if he was one of his totem animals disguised in a man's form. His feet seemed to barely touch the ground. To best honor what he taught, I will quote to you, as closely as I remember, the words he told us, over and over. It will be up to you, as it was left up to us, to see if you can find anything helpful in his words.

Support, support, support

"Support, support, support.

"If a patient is lying on the table, and you push down hard on them giving acupressure or massage, or push hard when you are feeling for the right place to put the hand or the needle, his body will automatically push back against you. There will be a fight going on. How can a person relax, how can he begin to heal, when he is fighting?

"If the patient is lying on his stomach, do not push his back down into the table. Instead, put one of your hands under his chest and your other hand on top of his back. Position the upper hand directly over your hand that is underneath. Now when you push on his back with your upper hand, resist that push with the hand that is underneath. That way, you are doing all the work; you are doing the pushing *and* the resisting. Your bottom hand is supporting the patient, holding him strong against the push of your upper hand.

"Support, support, support. You give the support; then the patient doesn't have to work at resisting you or work at supporting the weight of your hand. The patient can be peaceful, he doesn't need to resist you; you are resisting yourself with your opposite hand.

"The patient cannot relax if you are pushing or poking him. If your goal is to allow the patient to relax so that he can let go of his problem, do not hurt him. Give him support. Support, support, support.

"If you are going to have one hand on [some body part of the patient], your other hand should be on the other side [of the body part], catching the power of your first hand, protecting the patient from your active hand. If you are not doing any pushing, if you are just resting your hand on a patient, still, his body will have to worry about what to do about your hand. His body will be pushing back on your hand, especially if you are touching a part of his body that is scared.

"But if you support the patient by putting your other hand on the opposite side of his body [part] to support the patient, and use that other hand to catch the energy from the first hand, then the patient can relax.

"Sometimes both hands are active. Sometimes both hands are supporting. It doesn't matter. The only thing is this: the patient should not have to do *extra* work because you are imposing on him. The patient should be allowed to relax. Support, support, support."

Have fun

The master continued: "My attitude when I am giving treatment is that I am having fun. I learned that I gave the best treatments after I had already worked about eight hours. After working eight hours without a break, I start to feel hungry, tired. I cannot stay focused on my work even if I try. I begin to think that I cannot survive if I don't stop working. My mind becomes distracted from my work. I want so much to stop working that I cannot think about what I am doing. To keep myself going, I imagine that I am looking up at the blue sky. I imagine that I am at the beach.

"I love to go to the beach. When I go to the beach, I imagine that I am a red horse, a red pony, and I run in and out of the waves. When I am finished running in and out of the waves, I lay on the sand and look up into the blue sky.

"When I am starting to get so tired from treating clients, after about eight hours, but I can't stop because there are still more clients with appointments for several more hours, here is what I do: I think that I am lying on the beach, looking at the sky. I have discovered that during this time, when I am exhausted and looking at the sky, when the sky exists and the patient is no longer the center of my focus, *this* is when I begin to give good treatments. After a few more hours of still working hard giving treatments, when I am *in* the sky, when I *am* the sky, when the patient doesn't even exist anymore, then I am starting to do the best treatments. This is when patients get the best results. I learned this.

"So now, whenever I *start* working, I put my mind on the idea that I have already been working eight hours. I think that I can no longer keep going. I must start to imagine that I am looking into the blue sky. My idea is that I am so completely drained, I am so tired, I cannot think anymore about the patient. I can only survive if I am, in my mind, looking up at the sky with all my love and energy."

Shinzo-san often worked twelve and thirteen hour days without taking a break. His point, however, was *not* that he gave his best treatments at the end of a long day. His point was that he had learned that, no matter whether he was just starting his day or was starting on his twelfth client, his mind must always be as desperately seeking transcendent joy as a drowning man seeks for air. When he could hold his mind in this state, the treatments – no matter when they were scheduled – more or less took care of themselves. Meanwhile, what were his hands actually doing? Support, support, support.

Every week in shiatsu class, when he demonstrated his techniques on volunteer patients, I watched his hands. Where was he placing them? Very often he would start with the hands on the part of the patient's body that was having pain. But usually, as he gently pushed, vigorously pushed, or just let his hand rest firmly on the patient's skin - always with his other hand giving oppositional support – his hands would gravitate, with almost no conscious thought or motive, to some other part of the patient's body that seemed to want to be held, pushed, or prodded.

As his hands moved, patients would often blurt out something like, "I just remembered an old injury. It was just at the exact place where your hand is right now."

When he stopped thinking about what his hands were doing, his hands knew automatically just what to do.

Even if one of his hands then pushed or prodded, the patient never responded as if he was being pushed or prodded. The patient usually didn't seem to feel much of anything, except safety and relaxation, because the actual work of Shinzo-san's hands was somewhat undetectable to the patient's reflexive tendency to push back. Why? The support, support, support that his hands were giving each other.

Some of my fellow students resented this general talk about support, support, support. They kept asking him highly specific questions like, "Where's the right place to push on the patient for asthma?" or "What point should I push on for acid indigestion?"

They completely missed the point that the patient's own body would show you where the important blockages were. They deeply resisted the *fact* that the "curing point" for asthma or for indigestion is in different locations on different people. They wanted simple, one-size-fits-all location-formulas to cure the various diagnoses of their patients.

This formulaic focus on "curing points" is the reason so many patients don't get good results from acupuncture. (Please see my book, *Hacking Chinese Medicine*, for more on the subject of how acupuncture works, and why each person with a given set of symptoms might need treatment in a different location(s) than other people with the same symptoms. Available at www.JaniceHadlock.com)

I mention this, in part, because if you are looking for someone to do *Yin* Tui Na, you *cannot* assume that an acupuncturist, or even someone who is certified in Asian body-work, will necessarily be knowledgeable about or even *interested* in the "slow, hands-doing-the-diagnostics" style of FSR.

Control your thoughts

Another point that Master Fujimaki made was also very important, although I fear many of my fellow students only thought that he was relating a funny story.

"In Japan, we have a massage tradition that the patient leaves his clothes on. When I first came to this country, I was surprised that people remove their clothes for massage therapy. I was not used to working on bare skin.

"After I had been working in this country for about a month, I felt very bad about the way that my American patients behaved towards me. After every treatment that I gave, *every* treatment, the patient told me that he wanted to have sex with me. I thought that this was very bad. Young men, young women, old men, old women, they were all the same. After the massage, they all wanted to talk about having sex with me. I thought this was an American habit.

"One day I decided to learn why this was happening to me. I realized that I had a cultural difference about bare skin. To me, because of my Japanese background, bare skin suggested having sex. I must have been conveying my cultural ideas to the patients. So I made an effort to understand that in this country, bare skin was not a statement about having sex. I never again used this wrong idea about bare skin during massage.

Ever since that day, when I changed my attitude towards bare skin, not once after a treatment has finished has a patient wanted to talk about having sex with me, not *once*.

"When my mind was on sex, every patient thought about sex. Now I think about the red pony and the blue sky, and my patients think about whatever they want; and they recover from their pain and the sadness that was holding on to the pain."

I could write volumes about this shiatsu class that some, a few, students insisted taught us nothing, about classic shiatsu. However, I think the above examples make the two points most important to our work with patient's injuries or work with Parkinson's patients.

First, the patient must be supported. No matter how much or how little energy the health practitioner is applying to the patient's body, the patient should not feel the need to instinctively fight back or resist any of it. The patient should not need to push back unless he, for some reason, wants to. The support, support, support that Shinzo-san insisted on creates a pressure-free, supportive environment for the patient's body, as if the therapy, no matter how vigorous or how firm, somehow seems forceless *to the patient*.

The other important point is that the mental sojournings of the practitioner are important. The best results occur when the practitioner is not trying to give undue influence to the patient. If the practitioner's mind is focused on something, the patient can pick up on it and even misinterpret it.

Even focusing on healing the patient is usually inappropriate: if the practitioner is focusing on healing the patient and the patient is holding back for some reason, an unspoken conflict ensues. In the throes of this conflict, the patient cannot let himself go, he cannot relax. The patient cannot attend to the business of healing if he is busy fighting the practitioner or defending himself, however silently and invisibly.[1]

---

[1] This sentence sums up, very well, the problem that many patients are dealing with. *A person cannot relax and cannot let go if he is busy defending himself, however silently and invisibly.* Keep this phrase in mind as you work on your patient: do not judge him, do not try to mentally "help" him or pray for him. Mentally, *leave him alone.* Of course, you can always say prayers for him *after* the session is over and you are not technically working on him.

When the practitioner forgets about trying to heal the patient and plunges himself headlong into his own joy or inner peacefulness, the patient is less threatened. The patient can let his guard down. When this happens, the patient's body may very well start doing what it was designed to do: heal itself.

My class was the last year to have Shinzo Fujimaki as a teacher. The school administration, after receiving several complaints that: "Shinzo doesn't teach us anything *real*," replaced him with a dullard of a teacher who read to the students, right out of the standard texts, just where to push on various acupoints and how hard.[1]

Returning to the subject of "intention," Shinzo Fujimaki's work was most effective when he was focused on something other than the patient, such as being a red pony or gazing at the sky. The point he was making was "Mind your own business. Don't impose your hopes for your patient on the patient."

The following is a good example. A decade after taking his class, in one of the FSR clinics I taught, a student confided in me during clinic, "I feel like I'm not getting anywhere with this patient. He's Catholic, so I'm praying for Mother Teresa of Calcutta to inspire him and help him, but I just don't know…he's *so* rigid…"

I suggested that she forget about the patient and instead ask Mother Teresa to help her, the student, with her *own* problems.

She did so, and at the end of the class she reported to me, "I get it. The patient's skin stopped fighting me when I stopped trying to change him."

I have often beheld sudden, beneficial releases and tissue shifts in very "stubborn" patients while my mind was on highly mundane matters, such as compiling a grocery list. As for the idea of "correct intention," it might best be understood as "don't let your thoughts wander into negative areas, and keep your thoughts on something that is uplifting for *you*."

Dr. Paul Lee

Fulfilling another course requirement while I was still in school, I was privileged to take a class in Medical Qi Gong from a Qi Gong Master.

Dr. "Paul Lee" (Lee Pu Long), recently arrived from China, taught a brilliant class in which he taught us very specific techniques that patients could perform on themselves to stimulate their own healing energy in various body parts.

By way of introduction to Dr. Paul Lee, I will describe one of his projects. His work in China on self-applied eye "massage" had been adopted by the national government and was being taught to Chinese school children.

---

[1] Of course, this material was redundant. As second- or third-year acupuncture students, we already *knew* all the point locations and their applications. The replacement Shiatsu teacher simply demonstrated that these points could be stimulated by hand as well as via needles, and spent the whole semester doing it. I suspect that a few students liked this format because they didn't have to learn anything new. They could spend the class practicing acupressure on acupoint locations that they'd already studied.

I teach at an acupuncture college. *Most* students are highly idealistic, and want to do what is best for the patient. But I am including these "negative" bits to help the reader understand that, just as all MDs are not the same, all acupuncturists are not the same.

The government had wanted a solution to the problem of poor vision becoming rampant among children at the seventh and eighth grade level. As students were doing increasing levels of book-work, they were starting to need glasses. This is considered perfectly normal in the west, but in China, where the government is the supplier of eye exams and eyeglasses, this trend towards "student's myopia" was considered a health problem.

Dr. Paul Lee had devised a quick and easy program of Qi Gong (energy control) that included gentle finger stimulation of the bones around the eye socket *and* using the energized palms of the hands, held a short distance away from the eyes and then moved closer, further, closer again, over and over, to push and pull energy into and out of the eyes.

Starting in sixth grade, students did these quick exercises every day at school. They subsequently did not develop myopia and did not need glasses, even as they progressed through the later school years.

This type of Qi Gong exercise, in which the patient learns how to focus on a body part and move energy through it in a soothing, healing manner, is the essence of Medical Qi Gong.

This class taught me crucial lessons in the role that the patient plays in healing himself. If I could summarize the essence of the Qi Gong class, it would be this: the best doctor is one who sees where or what the source of the problem actually is, and then shares helpful information, even including specific exercises, to help the patient to change *himself*. The good doctor may advise on diet, exercise regimen, movement patterns, or instruct the patient in how to recognize where energy is moving incorrectly and how to correct it.

The point of the treatment is to help the patient learn what he was doing wrong that made him susceptible to the weakness or illness, and how to correct it. Ultimately, the responsibility for recovering and staying recovered is on the *patient*.

The job of the doctor is to non-judgmentally figure out the source of the problems in the patient and suggest to the patient a direction that will reverse the problem. The goal is relieving patient suffering through patient education and empowerment, which may include the patient learning some energetic (Qi Gong) exercises or learning an attitude adjustment. A further outcome is the confidence and positive attitude the patient develops as he learns how he can confront his own weaknesses and change them. [1]

---

[1] Regrettably, some western students of Chinese medicine have embraced a weird, ego-boosting version of "medical Qi Gong" in which the doctor uses his own energetic power to force healing onto a patient. While this may sound appealing to people who like the idea of having power over others, this type of work does not improve a patient's health in the long run. A patient who allows his body to be manipulated in this manner actually suffers a weakening of his own will power and his own sense of energetic control.

When the treated malady returns (and it will, sooner or later), the patient will be even less able to activate his innate healing energy than he was before. His body will passively wait for the next blast of healing energy from the healer rather than doing its own work. This type of healing, in which a charismatic person refers to himself as a Healer and forces the energy in a patient's body to move in an unnatural (not according to the patient's will) manner, is considered very bad form by many traditional Qi Gong practitioners. This type of work can be dangerous to the ego of the practitioner and does no long-term good to the patient.

Great souls from time immemorial have done miraculous healing work. However, these souls performed their healings by removing first the causal (ideational) problem that set in motion

Putting it all together

The many classes that I took in Asian and American bodywork, including some of the teaching in the Medical Qi Gong classes, all contributed to my understanding of Tui Na. Some of the techniques I learned in school had names. Some did not. The result of taking these classes, in addition to the other classes required for a Master's degree in traditional Asian medicine, was that I had learned, at least on a beginner's level, how to use my hands in a supportive manner.

When I got my license and started practicing medicine, if I did include Tui Na in the treatment session, I never bothered to mentally define which, if any, particular technique I was using on a given patient at any given moment of hands-on therapy. Everything I was doing was the sum of all the things I had learned. I suspect that this becomes true for all

---

the unhealthy energetics: the unhealthy energetics that manifest as the illness. Therefore, these great souls actually do remove the entire illness.

More importantly, they only perform these miraculous healings when their cosmos-attuned intuition tells them to do so. They have no personal desire as to whether the person heals or not at a specific time. For the most part, if they have a preference, they prefer that their patients seek the Truth and Love that will enable them, the patients themselves, to joyfully cast out their own health problems instead of passively waiting to be healed.

Patanjali, a contemporary of Socrates and one of the greatest Hindu writers on religious philosophy, makes this point in his Yoga Sutras. He explains that a sign of spiritual advancement is the ability to remove illness in another, including the underlying wrong thinking and past karma that caused the illness. But he also makes the point that a truly advanced soul may have this ability and, because of his wisdom, will choose the more difficult path: not using his spiritual powers to force an alteration in a person's chosen life direction unless commanded to do so by God. The truly wise understand the roles that sickness and health play in this worldly drama of cause and effect. The highest role, for a practitioner of medicine, is providing support so that the patient can heal himself.

However, some modern medical Qi Gong practitioners ignore this wisdom from the past. These well-meaning people, finding that they have the ability to temporarily alter a sick person's energy by physically or mentally manipulating their patient's energy, go ahead and do so, imagining themselves to be "spiritual healers." Even worse than the inevitable return of the illness in the original patient, these would-be healers often become deeply sick themselves despite their magic mantras, dramatic hand gestures, and bowls or gimcracks for "catching the bad energy." If this type of Medical Qi Gong healer does get sick, then when his "healed" patient's problem inevitably resumes, there are then two people sick with the same malady. From a larger standpoint, the world is worse off than before. Even if they do not get sick, these would-be healers are perpetrating the false idea that they, and not the patient's own self-directed life force, are the driving component of the healing process.

Only a Self-realized master can truly remove from the cosmos, through exercising his will in accordance with Divine instruction, the wrong energetics in another person's body, mind, and heart. However, each one of us has the right and the ability (usually undeveloped) to instantly or gradually heal ourselves from the results of our own wrong thinking, the wrong thinking that is our own source of our emotional, mental, and physical health problems.

In the new testament of the Bible, Jesus celebrated a teaching moment when he pointed out, insistently, that he was not responsible for the healing of the woman who clutched at his robe and was instantly healed. He emphasized that she, and not he, had worked the miracle. The miracle came about through *her* faith, through the change in *her* focus and thinking as she willingly tapped into the Love that Jesus personified. Jesus was trying to make the point that all of us have within ourselves the capacity for "miraculous" self-healing.

bodyworkers: at some point, one ceases to perform "techniques" and just "does whatever needs to be done."

When I started working with Parkinson's patients, I automatically sensed that I needed to use support, support, support to both assess their physiology and to treat it. Very possibly my own latent and utterly unsuspected Parkinson's symptoms, including my pathological aversion to being therapeutically "messed with" helped to guide me in this direction.

Putting FSR into writing

As already mentioned in the previous chapter, I only found out I was doing Yin Tui Na when I wrote my first article on Parkinson's and submitted it to the *American Journal of Acupuncture*. The editor told me that there was a generalized name for what I was doing: Yin Tui Na.

She also pointed out that Yin Tui Na was only a generic term, and for the article, she wanted to use a more specific name for the *exact* type of Yin Tui Na that I was using.

Then the editor paraphrased what I'd said by saying that the Tui Na I was using was a very light-touch, spontaneous-release type of Tui Na with no intention-based directional movement, which the patient *perceived* as forceless, as opposed to intention-based and perceived as forceful. I concurred.

So she had me refer to the Tui Na I was using as a Forceless, Spontaneous-Release style of Yin Tui Na, or FSR. She had me include in the article a few details about the FSR techniques I was using to make it very clear that the work was forceless to the *patient's* perception. The work was not directed at creating any particular response from the patient.

If, how, and when the patient responded, it would be some sort of spontaneous healing event on the part of the patient, not a change in response to anything *actively directed* by the practitioner.

The intent of the editor was not to create a trademarked technique. Nor was there an intention of implying that I had ever learned a specific, rarified technique of this name, passed secretly from master to master, through the ages. The editor and I were merely looking for a way to describe, as clearly as possible, exactly what it was I was doing. What I was doing was a Yin type of Tui Na, one that was *perceived* as pretty much forceless and intention-free, and which resulted in patients having some sort of release whenever they were ready to do so.

Again, I did not invent this technique. I learned everything I know from my teachers. They did not always have a name for everything they taught. My editor, rightly, wanted something more detailed than "holding," or "support" and came up with the adjectives "forceless" and "spontaneous release."

After publication, I was surprised by requests from people with Parkinson's looking for referrals for "FSR practitioners," as if FSR was some sort of "official" technique. At that time, I still considered it "simple holding," and only used the name FSR when writing about my Parkinson's research, in order to emphasize that the holding had to be perceived as forceless, non-intentioned, and that the releases, if any, would come spontaneously from the patient and not be "induced" by the practitioner.

By the time I web-published the fifth edition of *Recovery from Parkinson's* in 2000, even I was referring to the light-touch techniques I used on people with Parkinson's with the acronym "FSR." By 2012, when I wrote the edition before this one, I was so accustomed to the phrase "FSR," my mind's eye could see capital letters and an acronym where there used to just be two plain old adjectives and a noun. Somehow, this technique has turned into yet another named therapy!

But keep in mind, this is not a mysterious therapy from the misty past or the distant shores of Asia, but a simple method of using hands to work with an injured person. FSR is not a specific, exacting technique. FSR is just a way of providing support, support, support. Do not worry about doing it "correctly." Just do it, and enjoy doing it.

A frequently asked question:

Is there a Yin Tui Na practitioner in my area?

Again, there is no such thing as a *specific* technique called "Yin Tui Na," per se. "Yin," in this context, simply means, "on the gentle or 'light-touch' end of the bodywork spectrum." Seeking a "Yin Tui Na practitioner" is asking for a person who does *any* type of technique that is relatively gentle hands-on therapy, as compared to strong, vigorous therapy.

It does make sense to ask a practitioner who advertises "Tui Na" whether he has studied Yin-style or Yang-style techniques, or both. If the respondent says that he doesn't know, or if he says that he does "traditional Tui Na," this means that he probably has studied *only* Yang-type techniques.

Most people who study Tui Na in schools of Chinese medicine study only the Yang type. As a generality, while practitioners of Yin Tui Na are very aware of the existence of both the Yin and Yang kinds, many (most, in my experience) practitioners of *Yang* Tui Na are *not* familiar with the ideas of light-touch work.

People who *have* studied the Yin forms of bodywork have usually done so by studying western types of light-touch work. They would be more likely to refer to their techniques by the specific, western names of the particular modalities that they studied. For example, a western, hands-on, light-touch therapist might say: "I do both Gregson's cranio-tarsal work and Marco's Medical Unwrapping protocol," but he might have no idea that these light-touch therapies would be considered, in China, to be forms of Yin Tui Na.[1] Simply from lack of bilingual understanding, most practitioners of light-touch bodywork would probably *not* refer to their work as Tui Na. Many western-trained light-touch therapists have never even heard the term "Tui Na."

So the next question arises, "Is there a *FSR* practitioner in my area?"

Probably not. This is a pretty simple, dull technique. Few people get training in a technique of simple holding – a technique that any person can usually master in an hour or two.

So why do I stick with the fancy terms "Yin Tui Na" and "FSR"? Why don't I just refer to these techniques, in general, as "simple holding"?

I'm licensed as an acupuncturist. That license allows me to do therapeutic modalities that fit under the umbrella of traditional Chinese medicine – which, by California

---

[1] Both of these named techniques are fictional, created for the sake of example.

149

law, includes Tui Na. I am legally able to perform Tui Na. Officially, I am not licensed to "simply hold."

Also, no western terminology is as broad as the term Yin Tui Na. By using this term, I am giving myself the widest possible latitude in terms of techniques that are within the legal scope of my practice – even techniques that are as simple as providing firm holding with no expectations…techniques that *anyone* can easily learn to do, licensed or not.

Getting back to looking for a "trained FSR practitioner," you probably are not going to find anyone. These techniques, though utterly simple, have only recently been written up and given a name. Only recently have these techniques been discussed in the context of treating Parkinson's disease.

You probably cannot find *anyone* who is familiar with the name FSR unless he is already familiar with the research of the Parkinson's Recovery Project.

But the FSR techniques can be easily mastered by almost anyone who is able to sit still for several minutes at a time. You do NOT need to find someone who is "experienced" in this technique.

Become that person, yourself. You will find many opportunities to use this therapeutic work – and so long as you have your hands, you've got your tool kit with you.

Of course, if you really don't think you can do this type of therapy, or you really don't *want* to do it, you can share this book with your nearest craniosacral practitioner or massage therapist. If the first person you contact is not interested in doing this style of work, maybe he can refer you to someone who is.

Chapter nineteen

A proliferation of light touch therapies

This short chapter has been written because so many correspondents have told me that they feel nervous or even inadequate with regard to performing Yin Tui Na or, more specifically, FSR.

No matter how many times I write, "This is simple holding; a child can do it," I get frequent emails saying, "What if I'm doing it wrong?" or other phrases suggesting fear of failure to master the subtleties of this presumably tricky business.

I want to reassure every reader that, even if a light touch technique has a name, like "FSR," that doesn't mean it is necessarily technical, exacting, or needs to be studied under the auspices of some authority. And in the case of FSR, it's almost impossible to do it "wrong" unless you aren't holding firmly enough.

To help understand this, consider that many of the modern, light-touch techniques that can be placed under the broad umbrella of Yin Tui Na have their own, special names, even though many of them are based on very, very similar principles. In the vast panoply of light-touch therapies, it is sometimes impossible to say where one named technique leaves off and another begins.

In the last thirty years, it seems as if dozens, maybe hundreds, of therapists have been busy developing new "unique" versions of light-touch therapy and slapping their own names or a copyrighted trademark onto some variation of human touch. "Therapeutic Touch," "Unwinding," "Zero Balancing," "Bowen therapy," and "Upledger's craniosacral therapy" are just a few of the many trademarked or copyrighted "light touch" therapies that have been "created" or "invented" in the last few decades.

Some of these techniques claim to be unique because the hands are allowed to rotate a bit, compared to techniques in which the hands move in a linear fashion. Other techniques claim to be unique because the emphasis is on very short periods of touching or mere brushing against the skin, as opposed to touch that lasts for longer periods. However, for all these techniques, the underlying principles are universals, and not "inventions."

As an interesting legal point, techniques cannot be copyrighted. *Names* for techniques and the specific *text* used to describe them can be copyrighted, but, actually, the act of touching a person in a therapeutic manner *cannot* be copyrighted or patented.

For example (becoming a bit far-fetched, but hoping to make the point), holding a person's hand can be considered a form of hands-on healing. There are many ways to hold someone's hand.

An inventive person could, if he wanted, make up a specific name for the variation of hand holding that involves, say, interlocking the fingers. He could name this finger interlocking after himself and copyright that *name*.

This would *not* mean that this person discovered or invented the interlocked finger position. By law, he could *not* copyright the *technique:* he could *not* demand a royalty payment from people who interlock their fingers while holding hands. Nor could he prevent anyone else from writing about the technique of interlocking fingers – so long as that other person used his own words and a different name, if any, for the technique. Which is to say, so long as the other person does not plagiarize.

The inventive person could, however, publish books on the subject and hope that people would, from then on, choose to refer to themselves, whenever they interlocked their fingers, as doing the popular "Wilson Hold," or, depending on his name, of course, it might possibly be the "MacGruder Support" or the "Spongeworth-Hugeusson" Technique (if two people jointly wrote it up).

This self-glorifying labeling of body-work techniques might provide a person some temporary sort of name recognition and fame, and possibly some book sales. But just the same, a specific "technique" used while holding hands cannot be copyrighted.

Many of the "revolutionary" and "new" techniques that are flooding the field of light-touch therapy are, despite their copyrighted names, nothing more than the normal, intuitive touching and responding that emotionally healthy humans can do automatically – behaviors that are becoming more acceptable as our culture moves away from the rigid, "don't touch yourself or others" social rules of the past.

I am certain that if we modern humans, and even doctors (!), spent more time practicing touching our fellow humans in an intuitive, healing manner, the way that most of us easily and automatically rub, pat, and hold our pets, we would realize there is nothing new or particularly technical about the "miraculous" and "new" light-touch healing techniques that are so hot right now.

Not only that, I suspect that we *all* know how to do most of these techniques, already. Reaching out to one in pain is an innate function in most of the mammals. Weirdly, we humans are usually *taught* to not touch ourselves or others, according to cultural constructs.

But if we can overcome these "rules" that have been imposed on us, we find that we already know how to hold and encourage healing in others with our hands.

Since we modern westerners tend to *touch* very little and *feel*, or I might say *perceive*, even less, some, a few, members of the modern generations of would-be health practitioners might choose to take extra classes to learn *basic*, *core* medicine: how to touch, how to feel, and how to support with our hands. But most health practitioners, including MDs *and* acupuncturists, even after several years of medical school, have never learned how to touch and hold a patients' injured or insulted body parts in a supportive, constructive manner, let alone a diagnostic one.

Sadly, even after years of training, many health practitioners, both eastern and western, do not even know how to recognize which of a patient's maladies might best be treated by some type of hands-on therapy.

Fortunately, many of the researchers who are experimenting in this field are doing a brilliant job of writing about those techniques that work for them and publishing case studies. Of course, writing about this realm of light-touch therapy can be challenging: it can be just as difficult to describe in words just what a touch technique should feel like as it is to describe in words the flavor of an orange.

Still, many people in the field are working at making these light touch therapies better understood.

And many patients who have *not* responded to conventional western (allopathic) medicine have benefited from some of the new light-touch therapies.[1]

In English, we do not have a widely accepted medical umbrella term that covers all the schools of light-touch therapy. Therefore, they are each considered to stand alone – some even consider themselves as competing with one another. By referring to all the light-touch therapies as Yin Tui Na, by putting all of them under the same over-arching banner, it's easier to describe how the various light-touch techniques differ, and how they are similar. The differences, of course, can be as infinite as the human imagination and vocabulary allows. The similarity is that all these techniques employ the hands of the health practitioner in a supportive manner, in a fairly unobtrusive and/or somewhat undirected manner, in direct contact with the patient's skin or clothing.

But most important, and the purpose of this chapter's rant, is to assure you that *you* can easily learn do this work. It's just touching, holding, and supporting.

We're humans. Touching, holding, and supporting is *normal*.

That's it.

Whether a person is doing nothing but simple holding, or doing some of the "fancy" hand position holds of craniosacral therapy or the relatively quick, reflex-stimulating movements of Bowen work, the basic precept is *touch*, with, usually, some amount of supportive holding and, sometimes, fairly subtle movement, suggestions of movement, or even imagining movement.

Again, many of these simple techniques are *innate*. We see mothers with their babies doing these exact same techniques, automatically, to keep their babies comfortable and happy. When the infant is upset, the mother holds the baby snugly. When the infant is hurt, the mother kisses the spot and holds it, and at some point, starts to gently test the injured area. Sometimes, the mother gives just the lightest hug or jostle, at some tense spot, and the child's tension melts.

However, in many modern cultures, we are taught, at an early age, never to touch others except in specific, culturally approved ways. For many of us our innate understanding of how to hold the traumatized areas on another person's body has been squelched.[2]

---

[1] A study undertaken in the mid 1990s revealed, much to the astonishment of the allopathic medical world, that one third of the people in the US had used "non-traditional" medicine. The alarming thing was that a majority of these people had never told their doctors for fear that their doctors would respond with *anger*.

Of all the "alternative" modalities, acupuncture is the one most requested from people seeking alternative medicine coverage from their health insurance companies.

Hands-on therapies, including massage, are also very popular, but are almost never considered to be "medical." Unless the hands-on therapy is being done by a licensed Physical Therapist, it is usually dismissed as "feel good" treatment, and is not covered by insurance or deemed "significant" in resolving a biological problem.

[2] When I was attending high school in a highly urban area, I met a new student with whom everyone quickly felt very comfortable. If a classmate was stressed, the "new boy" would unself-consciously lay a comforting arm on a shoulder, or give just the right amount of pressure in a reassuring hand-hold. I was amazed at how he seemed to generate ease and comfort among

In learning the various forms of Yin Tui Na, and especially FSR, all we are really doing is relearning something that we already knew: how to give support with our hands in such a way that an injured or traumatized person can most quickly resume responsiveness and self-healing.

It's that simple. It's also extremely powerful.

A legal aside

At this point, you might be wondering why don't I refer to Tui Na as "bodywork" or "physical therapy" or, considering it's really just a type of normal holding, why don't I refer to it as "holding"?

Most acupuncturists are required to limit their treatments to their official "scope of practice." As a licensed doctor of Chinese medicine, I am allowed to perform – and bill – for treatments that are referred to as Tui Na. I am *not* allowed to perform or bill for treatments that are referred to as physical therapy or "supportive holding."

The actual treatment I perform might be exactly the same as that of a physical therapist, but from a legal and insurance point of view, under my licensing scope of practice, I must refer to my work as Tui Na.

On the one hand, this is an advantage to me. As a DAOM (Doctor of Acupuncture and Oriental Medicine, with as many years of training as an MD) in California, I am legally allowed to diagnose, prescribe, and treat. I get to figure out what treatment my patient needs and then apply it.

Most physical therapists must limit their therapies to those that an MD has prescribed.

Still, if *you* feel uneasy using a Chinese word to describe the therapies in this book, feel free to refer to Yin Tui Na as light-touch bodywork. The wording doesn't matter one bit, so long as you are not a licensed health practitioner. If you *are*, then it matters.

Acupuncturists in some states are required to take one or two classes in Tui Na to complete their degree in Asian or Chinese medicine. In many, if not most, acupuncture schools, the Tui Na classes teach only very *Yang* Tui Na techniques for specific bone displacements.

However, certifying laws in the states that allow a licensed acupuncturist to perform Tui Na never state what *types* of Tui Na he can perform. This means that a licensed acupuncturist may have studied only *Yang* Tui Na techniques in school, but he can legally perform craniosacral therapy, so long as he refers to it as Tui Na, which it is.

Craniosacral therapy is a light touch, Yin type of Tui Na (bodywork). Most acupucturists never learn to do craniosacral therapy in acupuncture school. If we want to learn it, we study it as "continuing education."

---

whomever he socialized with. I asked him where he was from. He was from a small rural area in Michigan. His family had kept dairy cows. Since his childhood, he'd spent his mornings and evenings among the cows. After I got to know his family, I realized that all of them had the same, slow, gentle, comforting way. He had never been trained in "light touch" therapy. He did it instinctively: he touched people the same way that he'd touched cows.

However, as an acupuncturist, one can bill insurance for a craniosacral treatment because it can be referred to as Tui Na, a form of Asian manual therapy. By definition, since craniosacral therapy uses the hands, it is a type of Tui Na.[1]

Officially, what is Tui Na?

If the hands of the practitioner make contact with the patient' skin or the patient's clothing, the practitioner is doing Tui Na.

When an MD in the emergency room repositions a patient's dislocated shoulder, the Chinese name for what the doctor is doing is Tui Na. When a chiropractor adjusts spinal bones, he is doing Tui Na. When a craniosacral therapist gently cradles the skull while feeling for the movement that pumps cerebrospinal fluids, he is doing Tui Na. When a shiatsu practitioner stimulates acupoints with his fingers, sometimes referred to as acupressure, he is doing Tui Na.

On the other hand, techniques such as Reiki, in which the hands hover over the patient but do *not* make contact, are *not* Tui Na. Energetic distance healing is not Tui Na. Techniques like acupuncture, moxibustion, or cupping, in which needles, moxa, or cups make contact, but the hands do not play a major contact role, are *not* Tui Na. Acu*pressure*, however, which is usually finger stimulation of acupressure points, *is* a form of Tui Na.

Between Yin and Yang

The difference between Yin and Yang techniques of Tui Na was discussed at the beginning of the book. However, some techniques are in the middle of the spectrum, not particularly Yang nor particularly Yin.

For example, Pediatric Skin Rolling, in which the supple skin of an infant's back is gently lifted away from the muscle in a rolling motion that travels from the skin near the neck down to the skin near the hips (or from the hips to the neck), is *mildly* active, inasmuch as the patient's skin is being actively moved. However, there are no particular bones, muscles, or tissues being targeted. This technique is neither extremely Yang nor

---

[1] The gross generality of referring, for acupuncture licensing purposes, to all hands-on bodywork as "Tui Na" leads to much confusion. Many people looking for a health professional to perform *Yin* Tui Na such as FSR for an injury or to treat Parkinson's disease have discovered that some health practitioners touting "Tui Na" on their websites very often have no idea that *Yin* type techniques even exist. When these practitioners studied Tui Na in school, what they learned was *Yang* Tui Na: powerful, body-jerking techniques.

For another example of confusion that arises by thinking that "Tui Na" refers to a specific type of bodywork, sometime around year 2000, in Texas, a judge suggested that Tui Na be removed from the scope of practice for acupuncturists. He was justifiably upset after seeing two cases, in one year, in which poorly trained acupuncturists had performed neck-cracking (chiropractic type) Yang Tui Na... and broke their patients' necks. The judge, not understanding that "Tui Na" means, essentially, "any hands-on therapeutic touch," wanted to make Tui Na illegal.

Technically, this would have outlawed all forms of touch on the part of acupuncturists, including feeling pulses (an action which, by mere contact, *can* slightly alter a patient's medical condition). I never heard the results of this attempt and have no idea what the current law is, in Texas.

extremely Yin, but is somewhere on the middle of the Tui Na spectrum – it might be called "mildly Yang Tui Na."

Acu*pressure* is another example of a hands-on technique that is not particularly Yang and not particularly Yin.[1]

Acupressure consists of gentle rubbing or pressing at the spot where some acupoint is located, in an attempt to stimulate channel Qi to move forward through an area that has insufficient energy flow. Like pediatric massage, it could be referred to as "somewhat-Yang" Tui Na. Then again, if the acupressure is somewhat subtle, it might be better described as "somewhat-Yin" Tui Na.

The psoas release technique presented in this book is mildly Yang inasmuch as it is an overt, visible, directed movement – but even so, it is very Yin in comparison to most other psoas release techniques.

All forms of hands-on body work, whether they were first written up in China, Sweden, or Beverly Hills, can be placed somewhere on the spectrum between Yang Tui Na and Yin Tui Na. In other words, "Tui Na" is not a term that refers to a specific technique for adjusting the neck or calming a frightened child.

All of the "new" *hands-on* techniques that are being "invented" as ways to therapeutically help a person address some illness or pain can be considered a type of Tui Na, according to the Chinese medical system. And, most of them can be easily mastered by *you*. FSR is probably the Yin Tui Na technique that is hardest to do *incorrectly*. There's really no way you can do harm while doing this technique. You can do it.

Why not give it a try?

---

[1] The word "acupressure" is a misnomer. "*Acu*" is from the Latin, and means "needle." The word "acupuncture" means "*puncture* with a needle." The word "acupressure" literally means "*pressure* from a needle," which it is *not*: it is pressure from a hand, or finger. It should be called manupressure or digipressure, or something like that.

Presumably, someone who had no idea that the prefix "acu" means *needle* came up with the word acupressure to describe pushing with fingers. The misleading word "acupressure" has come into common use, however.

Nothing to be done about it now, I suppose.

Chapter twenty

When and where to perform Yin Tui Na: a review

This closing chapter reviews the basics of Yin Tui Na techniques and of FSR techniques in particular. If you have gotten this far and still don't feel sure about the ABCs of how to start or how often to do treatments, this chapter will hopefully make it clear that you *do* know enough, and you *are* ready to start.

Some of this material is directed at acupuncturists. Most of it is general. The obviously redundant bits are addressing the most frequently asked questions.

Yin Tui Na techniques can be used to treat any physical injury, whether recent or old, in any patient. The exception is an injury in which some (non-broken) body part has been extremely dislocated and therefore *might* need strong, physical movements (*Yang* Tui Na) to be restored to its correct location. For example, a dislocated shoulder (when the ball of the humerus is out of its socket) might need to be physically muscled back into position. But less overtly displaced injuries may respond more quickly to the more Yin techniques of Tui Na. And even the large displacements might move more easily if the area is first treated with some type of *Yin* Tui Na, bringing relaxation and awareness to the area.

The three most common questions that arise at the acupuncture college where I teach are 1) *when* is Yin Tui Na indicated, as opposed to treating the patient with therapies such as acupuncture, herbs, laser, magnets, sound, and so on, 2) *where* is Yin Tui Na indicated, particularly in cases where pain at a certain location might be triggered by an unhealed injury at a *different* location. How can I determine the location of the root cause – and is that the place to perform Yin Tui Na, or should I treat the painful area and ignore the root cause? And 3) *how much* time, or how many treatments will be required to solve the problem?

When to perform Yin Tui Na on a patient

If a patient has pain that seems to be related to an *injury*, some Yin type of Tui Na is often a good first step in treatment/diagnosis.

The simple act of using one's hands on the injured area, with supportive pressure, will reveal whether or not the body part in question is *able* to respond in the normal manner.

If the patient's injured area yields a normal, reflexive response to supportive touch, Yin Tui Na is probably not *needed,* even though it might be pleasant and might accelerate the healing. But so long as there is normal responsiveness in the injured area, that area has the capability of self-healing.

In these cases, other therapies might reasonably be used to accelerate the healing, therapies such as acupuncture, physical therapy, light, sound, herbal therapies, a simple, cheap, ace bandage, instruction in the light and energy technique, or even just the passage of time might be all that is needed, depending on the injury.

However, if the patient's body does *not* perform a normal, reflexive response to supportive touch, it is very likely that acupuncture, physical therapy, and so on will *not* be particularly effective in dealing with this particular injury or trauma…yet.

If the patient's injury area has tissues that are broken or twisted and/or the micromuscle in the area is holding tight to prevent further injury, acupuncture or herbs will not necessarily reset the broken bone or unwind the twisted fascia. The micromuscle tension that is holding the injured mess in place will not necessarily loosen its grip in response to being attacked with acupuncture needles, cups, or lasers. However, the holding pattern *will* usually loosen up in response to human support that temporarily takes on the job of stabilizing and protecting the injured area.

When the patient's injured area is being protected and held immobile via the hands of the Yin Tui Na practitioner, the patient's body can relax its protective grip. The patient's body can then assess the injury or trauma, and begin healing it.

Only when the post-injury tension in an injured area is relaxed are any displaced or twisted body parts able to drift back to their correct positions. But when the area *has* relaxed, and the damaged bits have realigned themselves, these body parts can then commence any healing and reconstruction that needs to occur.

In almost any clinical situation where the patient has physical pain from injury, Yin Tui Na is appropriate. It might be FSR, or craniosacral work, or some other light touch therapy.

By the way, "light touch" does not mean "delicate." "Light touch" means paying attention to the patient's response. Light touch means not being overbearing.

Whether the pain is in a "tight neck" or sciatic nerve compression, there is nearly always some structural problem underlying the rigidity or pain. By "structural problem," I mean that some tissue, muscle, or bone has become somewhat displaced and/or is being held rigid by micromuscle. In most cases, acupuncture and/or herbs, alone, will not restore the displaced or tensed tissues to their correct and relaxed positions. Of course, once the structure is restored, then acupuncture, cupping, and/or herbs may be of great help. In most cases involving structural damage or displacements, the patient will heal much faster if some type of Yin Tui Na is used, initially.

For example, back pain usually responds to the stimulation provided by acupuncture, eventually. However, many visits are usually required to achieve full healing or even significant improvement. If the underlying structural displacements and micromuscle tensions are resolved *first*, and then the acupuncture is added to solidify the treatment, patients typically recover, or are significantly improved, in a mere one or two treatments, on average (based on my own clinical experience).[1]

---

[1] Studies abound regarding the efficacy of acupuncture in the treatment of back pain. In many of these studies, it appears that six treatments is considered about *average* for the resolution of back pain. To my mind, six is far too many treatments for an average. In my experience, the use of Yin Tui Na (usually psoas spasm release and/or some variant of a craniosacral protocol), prior to the acupuncture, can *greatly* reduce the healing time, even for *severe* back pain.

As an aside, it is unrealistic to make exacting estimates in a book, as to "how much" Yin Tui Na might be needed for treating the infinitude of possible back pain problems. In some cases, starting a treatment session with twenty minutes of Yin Tui Na, and ending with acupuncture, might be appropriate. In other cases, one or two sessions of nothing but craniosacral work, with possibly some psoas release work, might be best.

In long-term, severe cases, several sessions of nothing but simple, "boring" support might be needed to bring the body into some degree of correct structure, *after* which several sessions might be needed in which a few minutes are spent on some type of Yin Tui Na, with the rest of the time being used for acupuncture. If there is significant tissue damage, herbal treatment might be helpful, as well – once the basic structure has been restored.

In general, if there is any possibility of structural displacement, including bones, soft tissue, or even mental holding of micromuscle protection, treatment should begin with some type of Yin Tui Na and instruction in some techniques such as the light and energy Qi Gong in chapter five.

If, *after* structural irregularities have been treated, the channel Qi fails to revert back to its correct, parasympathetic flow patterns, then acupuncture might be used to restore correct channel Qi flow.

If the structure is restored and the channel Qi is once again flowing correctly, the body will be able to quickly heal itself. If significant amount of tissue damage occurred, herbs may be helpful in getting rid of the debris and swelling (referred to as Breaking up Blood Stagnation) and, later on, providing tonics for growing new tissues.[1]

The house building analogy

When building a house, the framing goes up first. Then the wiring. No one ever installs the wiring *before* the framing.

Doing "structural" repairs in the body are like working on the framing. These repairs often benefit from physical, hands-on therapies – Tui Na.

Doing mental Qi Gong is like getting mental "building permits."

Electrical repairs – fixing channel Qi aberrations – can be done using acupuncture and even herbs.

Sometimes, if there is no physical impediment such as scar tissue, the "electrical repair," which is to say the restoration of correct channel Qi flow, will resume automatically, following the structural repairs. In these cases, the Tui Na alone, with possibly some mental healing technique done by the patient, will have been sufficient to bring about both the structural repair *and* the electrical work.

Fix the framing before fixing the wiring.

---

[1] As a reminder to any acupuncture students reading this, remember that tonics should *never* be used so long as the injury is still in place. Breaks or displacement of the body's structural components constitute an "Excess" condition. We never use tonifying herbs or perform an acupuncture treatment that will bring more channel Qi into an area where there's already an Excess condition (including blocked Qi, Blood Stagnation or rebellious channel Qi). However, as soon as the underlying displacements ("Stagnation") have been resolved and correct channel Qi flow patterns have been restored, *then* tonification with herbs or needles might be helpful, especially in cases of extreme injury or constitutional weakness.

Broken bone example

If someone comes to you with a "compound" fracture (compound means that the broken bone is sticking out of the skin), you don't start treatment by inserting acupuncture needles in his arm. To do so would be like fixing a wiring problem without first fixing the broken framing.

It is obvious that, when someone presents with a compound fracture, you set the broken bones, first. Then, *after* the structure, or "framing" has been fixed up, or at least restored to correct position, *then* you work on restoring the disrupted energetic support to the area: you can then restore the correct flow of channel Qi by using acupuncture – if necessary. Again, in *many* cases, restoration of the correct positions of the structure allows the channel Qi to automatically resume its correct flow. If so, no acupuncture needling is necessary.

In the compound fracture example, the order for the sequence is obvious: fix the structural problem, *then* restore the energy flow to the area. The principle remains the same even when the structural component is far more subtle: frozen shoulder, a kink in the neck, ear ringing, foot pain. In all of these cases, the healing will occur far faster if the structural component is treated first. After the structural problem is resolved, the energy flow in the area can be corrected or amplified, if necessary, with acupuncture or with specific visualizations on the part of the patient.

Then again, because many patients go to see an acupuncturist expecting to get needles, it can be courteous to insert a few needles, whether or not the underlying structure has been completely restored, or even if the patient is still dissociated from the injury.

In such a case, choose to needle channels that are not affected by the obstruction, so that you will not make the error of "tonifying an Excess (injury) condition." Points such as Yin Tang (on the forehead), usually far removed from the point of injury, are usually harmless. However, to use *only* needles in a situation that would be far better treated with a combination of Tui Na and acupuncture is dereliction of duty.[1]

---

[1] I know acupuncturists who confidentially brag that they never "put their hands on" a patient. I know others who warn their colleagues, "Never do any hands-on work or body work of any kind. If you do any body work at all, the patient will enjoy it so much that they'll *always* want you to do it!"

Some practitioners have a snobbish attitude against using their hands: they consider that acupuncture is more sophisticated; Tui Na is a "lower class" type of treatment.

Others have financial reasons for disdaining hands-on therapies: you can only treat one patient at a time if you're doing Tui Na; you can treat six patients an hour if you never do anything but needles and you let your interns do the moxa and take the needles out. Sad to say, I know *teachers* of acupuncture and Asian medicine who propound these needle-only beliefs and attitudes.

Happily, in my own few decades in the field I have seen an increase in the number of practitioners who appreciate that the patient's needs come first. These practitioners, who provide the slow, time-consuming Tui Na if necessary, also generate an extremely high degree of customer loyalty. In my own practice, I've had patients who've temporarily used other acupuncturists when I've been out of town. They come back to me as soon as possible, with remarks such as, "He never even *felt* my neck to assess the painful place," or "She didn't pay any attention to *where it hurt*! She just stuck needles in!"

Puzzled acupuncture students often wonder why their theoretical studies don't lead to treatments that really do the job. Very often it's because the treatments they observe, and perform, in

Summarizing *when* to use Yin Tui Na

If you are a lay reader, planning to help friends or family members by performing Yin Tui Na techniques to help support an injury, you don't have to worry about what other options, such as acupuncture, *might* be helpful. However, if you are a health practitioner, you must be able to decide what kind of treatment(s) will be best for each individual.

In California, an acupuncturist might be trained to carry many tools in his kit: herbs, acupuncture, Tui Na, dietary counseling, or energetics (Tai Qi, Qi Gong, visualization, etc.). What is not taught, enough, is deciding *which* of these tools to use on a given patient or ill-health presentation.

Of course, we learn in school that the age and constitution of the patient, as well as the nature of the problem, will help determine what type of therapy is used.

For example, young children and infants are nearly always treated with gentle, skin-rolling Tui Na, and almost never given strong acupuncture needling. Very old people also benefit tremendously from the human touch of Tui Na, prior to any needling. When working with pregnant woman, you should use Yin Tui Na and needle "mild" acupoints. If stimulation at one of the stronger, "Qi-shocking" acupoints, such as LI-4, is called for, we might use very gentle acu*pressure*, instead of needling.

Even so, some students graduate with the idea that, in general, acupuncture should always be tried first, and the other options should be used only if the patient doesn't respond after many, many acupuncture treatments. These students have often forgotten one of the first rules of Chinese medicine: "Never tonify an Excess condition."

---

a college of Asian medicine, are designed to develop their *acupuncture* skills and their familiarity with the classic "illness patterns" related to herbal medicine. By learning this material, they are most likely to pass the licensing exam, a noble goal. *But* acupuncture and/or herbs might *not* actually be the best treatment for the patient's needs.

Very often, injured or traumatized patients will benefit more from Tui Na, prior to or instead of acupuncture. Without Tui Na, the patient may *not* heal as quickly. As for the Shen disturbance aspect (mental/emotional trauma, dissociation, pause, and so on) of a serious injury, this can often be best addressed by the mental medical Qi Gong exercises in chapters five and six of this book. Failure to do this might lead to slower healing – if any.

However, this mental aspect of therapy is utterly ignored in many training clinics, even more than is Tui Na. The primary focus in many schools of Asian medicine is acupuncture. This is understandable: the primary focus of the schools *must* be training their students to pass the acupuncture board exams. Tui Na and medical Qi Gong are *not* usually included on board exams, which vary from state to state.

Very often, at colleges of Asian medicine, most of the faculty is highly trained in acupuncture, and not particularly comfortable with performing Tui Na. Sadly, many schools have *one* academic teacher to teach the required Tui Na class, and *one* academic teacher for the required massage class.

Meanwhile, the *clinic* (non-academic) instructors are acupuncturists who often have little or no interest or proficiency in body-work. So even if the students take a few classes in bodywork, they rarely have a chance to observe it in clinic, or practice it on their patients under the clinical teacher's protective eye. As for mental medical Qi Gong, it is rarely taught, and almost *never* used in training clinics.

The above is not intended to put acupuncture schools in a bad light – it is merely to serve as a warning that a licensed acupuncturist may not be very experienced in Tui Na or Qi Gong unless he has gone out of his way to study it, usually in post-licensing continuing-education classes.

Injury, encoded in Chinese medicine as "Blood Stagnation," is *always* an "Excess" condition. In nearly every case, inserting a needle into some acupuncture channel will increase – tonify – the flow of Qi in that channel. If the Qi is running backwards, the needle insertion will increase the power of the backwards flow. If your patient feels a ferocious electrical jolt and breaks into a cold sweat, it is highly likely that you have needled into a channel that was severely blocked or running backwards…and you have just made his situation worse.

If you want to avoid violating one of the most basic precepts of Chinese medicine, the rule to "Never tonify an Excess condition," Yin Tui Na is very often the first modality of choice *any* time that tissues, including muscles, bones, tendons or ligaments, or even organs, are displaced.

Yin Tui Na can also be used for other types of problems with an *injury origin*, such as headaches, vision and/or hearing problems, sinus problems, stiffness, digestive problems, and numbness, to name a few. In all these examples, the underlying root cause might be injury, spasm, or structural displacement – Excess conditions, all.

On the other hand, if the patient's problems are being caused by pathogens (Evil-Wind), toxins in the diet, stressful climatic conditions (Cold, Heat, or high humidity, also known as Damp), emotional tension (Liver Qi Stagnation) mental disturbance (Shen disturbance), scar tissue (Blood Stagnation) or any of the other, *non*-injury root causes, an approach other than Yin Tui Na might be better. The health practitioner *must* diagnose the root of the illness in order to know which treatment modality to use.

Yin Tui Na can also be helpful if a patient is trying to consciously rid himself of emotional (Shen disturbance) problems brought about by any of the seven "Pernicious Emotions": fear, anger, melancholy, anxiety, excess sadness (self-pity), worry, hysteria, and fright (panic). The hands-on support of various forms of Yin Tui Na, *combined* with mental medical Qi Gong, can sometimes be extremely effective.

People with emotional traumas buried in their past very often hold tension in their neck, lungs, diaphragm, liver or heart area, to name just a few holding spots. By applying hands-on support to these and other soft tissue areas, a therapist using Yin-type Tui Na methods can often initiate healing of problems such as asthma, insomnia, indigestion, or other maladies and pains, *if* these problems were stemming from traumas being retained in structural displacements or in twisted soft tissue – so long as the patient is also working on changing the mind-set that allowed the tension to be retained.

Yin Tui Na, *combined* with mental medical Qi Gong is probably *the* most effective clinical means of treating a disorder in which the patient has mentally *dissociated* from the trauma. If the patient has dissociated, no number of needles, no number of herbs, will break through the mental barrier formed by the patient.

Where to perform Yin Tui Na on a patient

How do you locate the place on the patient's body where you will begin your application of Yin Tui Na?

Of course, if a patient complains of ankle pain after recently turning his ankle, you will put your hands on the ankle area. If he's recently broken his radius, you'll hold his arm at the point of fracture. These are the easy ones.

162

But patients often insist that there has been no injury at all, or no injury in the problem area. Sometimes, the patient has just forgotten the injury. Other times, the patient dissociated from the injury, and cannot remember it. Sometimes, the pertinent injury is not mentioned because the root injury was in a different part of the body from the current pain, and the patient doesn't see any connection – hence no reason to mention the significant injury.

Very often, the place that hurts is *not* the same place as the injury that lurks at the root of the problem. For example, sciatic pain in the ankle or leg may arise from tension in the hip area (putting pressure on the sciatic nerve) in order to hold the body fairly rigid…so as to protect a forgotten or now painless *neck* injury. I have seen a case of sciatica in which the left-side hip and leg pain was set in motion by a blow to the right-side back of the head.

Ear ringing *usually* has its origin halfway down the body…in a psoas muscle spasm in the lower half of the spine that is triggering a compensating twist in the temporal bone (the bone through which the ear canal is located) on the opposite side of the body.

As another example, frequent sprains in the ankle along the Gall Bladder channel may have their origin in a *head* injury along the Gall Bladder channel, a head injury that's causing deficiency (weakness) along the length of the channel, but only showing up in the weak ankle. Then again, frequent ankle sprains might have their origin on the Stomach channel.

And dystonia in the arm and shoulder on one side of the body can be set in motion by protections of an injury from the *opposite*-side arm and shoulder.

Yet another example is the manner in which problems in the vicinity of Ren-1 or Ren-2 (the Ren channel flows up the middle of the front of the torso) may be the result of injury, long ago, at *Du*-26 (the Du channel flows up the back). After all, the Du and Ren channels mingle during their internal passage down the gastro-intestinal tract, and a glitch in one of these two channels can cause a corresponding glitch in the other one, which manifests when the channels emerge from the anus and begin, once again, their flow towards the head.

Given that just about any injury, if unhealed, might trigger compensations nearly anywhere in the body, how can one possibly hope to know where the keystone injury, the basic, underlying, root cause, is located?

As an aside, I realize that some of the above may seem obscure, or off-topic, for the person who simply wants to learn Yin Tui Na in order to treat the feet of a friend with a twisted ankle or treat someone with Parkinson's disease. But by including these few extra examples this book can be a more complete text for acupuncture students, whose patients might present with an infinite array of problems.

Where to begin treatment

Very often, the patient's pain or problems are not in the same location as the unhealed injury. Many people with Parkinson's have neck stiffness or hip pain, but the root cause might be unhealed foot or ankle injury. Until you treat the root cause, the other pains and problems will not go away for good.

Some approaches to Yin Tui Na treatment address this unknown-location problem by treating as broad an area as possible, on the assumption that, by treating everything, you're bound to hit the problem area, as well.[1]

For example, most schools of craniosacral therapy teach a multi-step protocol in which every bone in the cranium, spine, and pelvic girdle, plus a few of the ribs and the clavicles, are supportively held, however briefly. This approach is moderately *thorough*, but also causes much time to be somewhat wasted – time that might have been better used by directing one's attention to the exact, specific location. Then again, by touching a large range of locations, the main location of injury and the subsequent compensation areas are *likely* to be all addressed during one session. If you aren't able to discern the root location, the site of the original unhealed injury, it's reasonable to take the sweeping view and touch on as many areas as possible during the first or second session with a patient.

Many practitioners who've done craniosacral therapy for many years eventually realize that, in any given patient, they only need to focus on a few of the holding positions – the areas that have no response or only a very weak response. But they learn this only after some hands-on experience – or else by learning, right from the beginning, how to recognize when responses from a specific body part feel "right" or feel "wrong."

An important diagnostic tool

Some very simple ways to determine whether or not the patient has constructed a mental barrier, and if so, *where*, are in the diagnostic protocols in the appendices of this book.

One of them, for example, explains that you might ask the patient to imagine light and energy in some healthy part of his body (the tip of the nose is *usually* a safe spot, unless there is a history of injury to the head). Then you ask the patient to imagine the same amount of light and energy in the rest of his body. If the patient finds an area that is dimmer or less able to be illuminated and energized, that area might be a good place to start.

If you know where the exact location of the injury is

Even if you know where an exact "point of injury" is, that place might not be the *only* location that needs treating.

Continuing to use the example of craniosacral therapy, sometimes a patient knows exactly where the injury occurred, but it's no good to just treat that location. For example, a

---

[1] For students of Asian medicine, be aware that pulse diagnosis will probably not help you know *where* the root of the problem, the unhealed injury, if any, is located. For that matter, as most students of Asian medicine quickly learn, despite the assurances of their theory classes, a person with pain from physical injury (a form of Blood Stagnation) does *not* necessarily have a wiry pulse, just as a person with a wiry pulse does *not* necessarily have pain from Blood Stagnation. For that matter, a person who has dissociated from his injury or is on pause is likely to have a very deep, almost un-findable pulse – the very opposite of the "wiry pulse" that theoretically accompanies injury or pain.

As for tongue diagnosis, Blood Stagnation from injury is only rarely reflected on the tongue. Many people with what you'd call "Blood Stagnation from unhealed injury" or Parkinson's have perfectly normal tongues and tongue coats, or their tongues reflect some other condition unrelated to the unhealed injury.

person who falls backwards on his head may know perfectly well that his injury occurred to his occipital bone. However, the force of the blow may have caused displacements or twisting in his other cranial articulations, his cranial fascia, his neck, and even his lower spine. The force of the blow to the occipital bone will probably have traveled to the front of the face, particularly the sphenoid bone, and may have traveled into the neck, particularly the upper cervical vertebrae. From there, the force of the blow may have also become distributed to the frontal bone, the temporal bones, down the spine to the lumbar vertebrae, and into the sacro-iliac joint.

In a case like this, the practitioner will want to give support, and the opportunity of restoration, to all of the affected bones and soft tissue. In this case, even though the injury was highly localized, performing an entire craniosacral protocal, touching on all of the areas with repercussions from the injury, will best meet the case.

Which still leaves the question open: how do we know where to start applying Yin Tui Na, if we don't know exactly where the pain or problem started?

Use Tui Na to find areas that don't respond

Using FSR diagnostically was discussed in an earlier chapter: by learning how a healthy body part responds to supportive touch, and learning to recognize the unresponsiveness or incorrect responses of an unhealed, injured area, an FSR practitioner can hold the patient's body in many locations, testing for responsiveness. By spending a few moments in many locations, he can quickly zero in on the area or areas at the root of the problem – even if the root is at the opposite end of the body from the patient's pain.

Even if the area with an abnormal response is only a "branch" of the problem, and not the root area, treatment of the branch very often leads the practitioner's hands to move, intuitively, quickly, to the root. Performing FSR and "listening" to the signals coming from your intuition can be an excellent way of knowing where support and holding, or some other type of Yin Tui Na, is needed.

Feel the flow of channel Qi, looking for aberrations

Another skill is feeling for errors in the flow of channel Qi. The location of a glitch in the flow of channel Qi suggests an underlying problem at that location – even if there is no obvious pain coming from that area. Knowing how to feel channel Qi, directly, by hand, can be of enormous benefit when looking for an unknown root cause. Once a person has mastered the easy-to-learn art of feeling the actual channel Qi flow, he can assess the patient's entire body in under five minutes.[1]

---

[1] Learning how to feel the flow of the sub-dermal currents by hand is taught in *Tracking the Dragon,* a textbook on advanced channel theory. Written originally for acupuncture students, it is also accessible to people with *no* medical background. The book is available at www.JaniceHadlock.com.

Hacking Chinese Medicine, a breezier, more introductory book on general Chinese medical theory and terminology, is also available at this website.

Learn the most common compensating mechanisms

Another skill set that can help in determining the location of the root problem is memorizing the most *common* compensating mechanisms. These most common compensations account for a majority of the problems seen in clinic. A few of very common situations in which pain is perceived in one part of the body but has origins elsewhere was already mentioned earlier in this chapter: sciatic (hip and leg) pain from head injury; ear ringing from psoas spasm (lower torso); and ankle weakness from neck bone displacements.

To find the actual starting point of a person's pain, you may need to be a bit of a Sherlock Holmes, because the possibilities are infinite. But if you trust your hands and your intuition, you will often be quickly guided to the place that "really doesn't feel right."

How long before the injured body part responds to FSR treatment?

How many treatment sessions will be required?

This technique can work very quickly, within minutes, for a very recent injury (in the last twenty-four hours).

Oppositely, with injuries that have been ignored for decades, and particularly if the patient, at the time of injury, *decided* to deny the pain and injury (self-induced dissociation or self-induced pause), the injury might not release for weeks, months, or years (assuming one-hour treatments once a week).

I had a Parkinson's patient whose utterly rigid feet received three years of intermittent FSR therapy, with approximately fifteen to twenty treatments a year, with no apparent response. Until, during one session, he was suddenly able to move his ankle, wiggle his toes, feel his feet, and all other normal foot functions. His chronic foot pain and immobility disappeared. After that, he was once again able to find shoes that "fit right." His ability to play tennis returned. The changes in his "frozen" right foot occurred in a matter of minutes.

On the opposite side of the time-frame spectrum, a person with a recently (in the last 24 hours) broken bone may respond to FSR within minutes – even if the bone has already been somewhat set and is already encased in hard plaster.

Broken bones: an aside

Even if a broken bone is already encased, application of FSR, with supportive hands resting on the *outside* of the plaster or plastic cast, can allow the twisted tissues inside the cast to relax and "reset" themselves, perfectly. If the injury was very recent, the injury can often be restored to health within minutes. It is very rewarding. It can also be perceived as "miraculous" by the patient, who can usually feel the bones moving around "spontaneously" inside the hard cast.

In these cases, it becomes clear that the electromagnetic support from your hands is doing as much, or more, than the actual physical contact of your hands.

This technique can help the broken ends of the bone realign themselves *perfectly*. This perfect alignment is similar to the way in which broken porcelain can be set back together so exactly that the seam is invisible, and a faint electrostatic bond between the porcelain pieces tentatively holds the pieces into place.

When this perfect reset can be brought about in a broken bone, through the use of FSR, the broken bone often stops hurting, the tissues around the bone stop hurting, and healing can be extremely rapid.

I've known patients (patients who did *not* dissociate from the pain) to be able to walk on a broken foot or ankle bone in three days, with no casting, by having received FSR treatment within several hours of the injury.

Toes and collar-bones

Typically, a western doctor will not bother to reset a broken toe. Even with a broken collar-bone (clavicle), the doctor often just puts the arm in a sling and doesn't reset the collar-bone itself, unless the bone parts are significantly displaced. These injuries are usually left to "heal themselves." They rarely heal correctly. The toe or collar-bone may be torqued, and a source of pain, for the rest of the patient's life. If you can treat such an injury within a few days of the injury, before the break has begun to knit with an incorrect alignment, you can use FSR to help the bone ends restore themselves to their exact correct position, and save the patient from a lifetime of nagging pain.

When bones "refuse" to knit

Also, in cases of a bone that has been casted but has failed to knit, even after one or two periods of the typical six-week wait, application of FSR can support the injured area so that the area relaxes enough to eliminate the twisting in the soft tissues that was keeping the bone ends apart, and releases the static forces in the tissue that remain as a result of the injury. As soon as these forces are resolved, the ends of the bones revert to their original positions, bringing the broken edges close together in a perfect fit. Once this occurs, knitting of the broken ends commences immediately, even in bones that had been failing to knit.

If the patient is wearing a cast, place your hands on the cast and leave them there. Remember, you are not so much pressing on the *patient* with your hands as you are mentally pressing your two hands against *each other*. An electrical field will quickly develop between your two hands, passing through the cast.

Soon enough, the patient will feel "something going on" in the vicinity of the break even though you are not touching the patient's skin. The patient's attention, and even his subconscious, will be drawn to the area, and the field generated between your hands will make the injured area feel safe, as if it is being held. The patient will probably feel his muscles relaxing and unwinding inside the cast, and might even be able to feel the bones moving back to their optimal position.

Of course, if the emergency room or orthopedic MD has made things trickier for you by putting a few "pins" in the bone to hold it in place – without first having released the tension in the surrounding soft tissue – it may be nearly impossible to help the bones reset themselves. The tension in the soft tissue, together with the tension that the physician introduced to the tangle, *all held in place by the pins*, can sometimes prevent the bone from knitting quickly and easily, and no amount of FSR will be able to get rid of those pins. If you can get the surgeon to remove the pins, you will have a much better chance at helping the patient heal completely, especially in those broken bone cases that exhibit "failure to knit."

In my own practice

As an acupuncturist, I use FSR for people with problems ranging from chronic headaches to kidney stones. I *very* frequently use craniosacral techniques and the psoas release taught in this book. They are simple but powerful tools that can be used by health practitioners and people with no background in medicine.

My formal training is in Chinese medicine. The field of Chinese medicine includes Tui Na. In my medical practice, if the patient's problem is one of stiffness, numbness, pain, or injury I almost always start the treatment with Yin Tui Na, not acupuncture.

Actually, I usually start by feeling the flow of the channel Qi over the entire body, figuring out where the energy isn't moving correctly. Then, by asking more questions, I try to figure out the history: *why* the energy isn't moving correctly. Once I have a workable and plausible hypothesis, I will often try Yin Tui Na at the most likely *initial* location of the problem. I will also usually ask whether or not the patient is able to visualize the area where the energy is *not* flowing.

After all, my job is not to heal, but to find out *why* the patient is not healing.

If the patient is dissociated, has self-induced dissociation, pause, or self-induced pause, I will help the patient work on those mental situations.

If the patient's electrical currents are just "stuck," I will *usually* start with Yin Tui Na to get him "un-stuck"... unless there is scar tissue that is blocking a critical part of the subdermal electrical system, in which case I will *usually* start with acupuncture on the scar(s).

If, after all the body parts have normal responses to FSR but the channel Qi is still not moving, which is rare, I will *usually* use acupuncture to stimulate the flow of channel Qi that has become mis-routed.

I have included this short bit on my own professional approach to make the point that acupuncture and "fancier" protocols are very often *not* necessary.

In your own practice

So here you are. You know everything you need to know to get started.

You hold in your own hands a collection of tools that you can use to help your friends, your loved ones and, if you are a health care professional, your patients.

I hope, by now, you are throbbing with confidence.

Be sure and practice a bit of holding and letting go on a healthy person before you work with someone with injuries.

Ask permission.

Settle in, get comfortable, and supportively hold another human.

Notice what you feel, but don't try to influence what happens under your hands.

Trust your hands and your intuition.

You are ready to start.

Appendices

The following two appendices were lifted, with modifications, from chapters in my book *Stuck on Pause* (available for free download at www.pdrecovery.org).

The first appendix addresses dissociation and self-induced dissociation.

The second appendix addresses pause and self-induced pause.

They are included here to help people determine whether their health condition is possibly being held in place by some sort of mental denial or is biologically stuck due to not finding a safe time and place to address a past trauma.

Techniques for treating both types of dissociation are included in chapters five and six of this book.

Treatment for pause and self-induced pause is included in the book *Stuck on Pause*, available for free download at www.pdrecovery.org.

Appendix I

Diagnosing dissociation and self-induced dissociation

Before receiving Yin Tui Na treatment, you will want to determine if you are dissociated, using self-induced dissociation, stuck on pause, or using self-induced pause.

This appendix and the next can help you figure out what mental blockages you have created, if any.

Please note, *not* every one with a chronic health problem has dissociated from the area or is on pause. In my own practice, I've seen that *most* people's *chronic* problems are due to something more physical and not so much mental. Only when the usual illness factors are ruled out and the problem would normally be expected to have healed long ago, *or* the channel Qi keeps running incorrectly for no apparent reason and does not respond to traditional treatment *or* only responds temporarily, do I start to consider that the patient might be using his mind to hold his health problem in place.

With my own patients, I have noticed that the more a person is capable of strong mental focus and analytical thinking, and is word oriented rather than somatic sensation oriented, the more likely he is to have a mental holding pattern in place.

What do you see?

If I even suspect a patient might be dissociated from some body part or on pause, I want to know what he sees when he visualizes – or fails to visualize – what's going on inside his body. Can he imagine, inside his own body, bright, cheerful light, deep darkness, or something in-between? Which locations for light or dark areas does he find? Is it *easier* to see light or *easier* to see darkness in various parts of his body, especially parts that might be having health problems or a history of injury?

Start at the nose

If I think that there might be some mental factors preventing or slowing the healing process, I usually start by asking the patient to visualize white light in the tip of his nose.

Most people, even if they have dissociated from some limb or torso area, are still able to imagine light in their *nose*. Of course, if they have had a broken nose or a nose surgery, they might not be able to do this. In these rare cases, I choose another presumably neutral starting point such as the chin or an ear: some small area close to the head with presumably no history of injury, scarring, or pain.

I start by asking the patient "Can you close your eyes and imagine a bright light in the tip of your nose? If he says no, I ask if he can imagine the inside of his nose being *dark*? Or I might say, "Which is easier, light or dark?"

If the person says, "Yes, I can imagine bright light [or darkness] in my nose" (or whatever neutral starting point he's using), I then ask him to imagine light in some finger.

If he can't imagine either light or dark in his nose, I try various other body parts. If the person is on self-induced pause or self-induced dissociation from his entire body, he might not be able to imagine any light or dark *anywhere*. The imagination part of his brain may be set to "risk" mode, a situation in which a person is usually only allowed to imagine negative outcomes, and very often cannot do visualization with regard to his own body. This situation is far more likely to result from pause than from dissociation. We'll get back to this.

After visualizing light or dark in the nose, or some other neutral place, if the person's suspected injury or trauma is on the *left* side of the body, I next ask the patient to imagine light or dark, whichever is easier, in his *right-side* index finger – on the untroubled side. If the problem is on the left, I ask him to imagine light or dark in the *right* finger.

If the index finger has scarring or signs of weakness, such as fungus under the fingernail, I choose some other finger or the thumb.

In these beginning, testing enquiries, the patient is working at increasing his confidence in being able to visualize. It doesn't really matter *what* he imagines he is seeing.

Then, after he has successfully imagined light or dark – whichever is easiest – in a few places that are *not* the main problem areas, I ask him to keep his eyes closed and imagine light or dark, whichever is easiest, in the vicinity of the problem area.

If the person has *dissociated* from some part of his body, this body part may be very hard to imagine as being full of light but it may be very easy to imagine as being dark, shadowy, or cloudy. Sometimes, it is dark to the point of non-existence. That's fine.

Very often, the person interprets the darkness as proof that the body part is badly damaged. This is wrong.

The darkness is not coming from the body part. The darkness is a purely mental construct. It's the *brain* that not being able to imagine light, or maybe anything, in this area.

If unable to imagine light in the area, the person is NOT actually *seeing* trauma or the damage in the area. His *brain* is refusing to *imagine* anything, or at least anything positive, in the area. (See drawing, page 26.)

I repeat: when a person imagines light in some part of the body, he is merely playing a visualization game – the person isn't actually seeing the inside of that body part. What he's seeing, in his mind's eye, is how he *feels* about that part of his body – whether or not he's even able to *think* about or have somatic awareness in that part of his body.

When he sees darkness, he's *not* actually *seeing* that the area is lacking in life or light. He's seeing that his *mind's access* to that area is fully or partially blocked off.

Doing a whole-body scan

Sometimes, a person has so many injuries and/or health problems that he has no idea where in his body to begin imagining light and dark. In such a case, he might choose to be methodical. He can start at one extremity (the toes or the fingers) on one side of the body and try to mentally imagine light or dark in one area after another, spreading out from the starting point. Or he can start at the head and work his way down to the feet.

Another instruction I might use is "Mentally look for the body part that you *most* don't want to look at." Or "Mentally look at the area that tightens up or feels yucky when you're nervous or emotional."

Once the person finds an area that's dark, darker than the rest or *more* invisible than the rest, I ask him to do the next step: focus on the darkness and try to notice if the area is immobile or agitated.

Motionless

If the dark place has is an *absence* of movement, an absence of the feeling of life itself, or the body part in question is missing altogether, the darkness is probably due to dissociation. If the area is dark and *heavy, motionless,* or *non-existent*, it is very likely that the person either automatically dissociated during some trauma and never got around to re-associating *or* he consciously instructed himself to dissociate from the area.

In either case, he will probably remain dissociated until he takes steps such as the re-association exercises in chapters five and six and/or gets therapy (including therapy such as FSR) to turn off the dissociation. If he does both, doing mental exercises and getting physical support, the dissociation might get turned off much more quickly.

Agitation

Oppositely, if the dark area is agitated or *moving* in any way, the person is probably using *pause*, not dissociation, in that part of the body.

People who are stuck on *pause* due to a near-death trauma or a decision to feel no pain will likely see a dark area that seems to be vibrating, trembling, or somehow agitated. Indications of pause will be discussed more in the next chapter.

Dark and still in the center

Sometimes the imagination can put a thin veneer of light over a dark area.

If *you* have a chronic problem area that *appears*, to your imagination, to be filled with light, but you suspect that the area is in fact dissociated, look at the very *center* of the problem area. The very core center might be large, or it might be as small as a pea, or smaller. A dark area might be haloed with light on the perimeter, but looking at the very center of the problem area might reveal darkness at the center.

After a person finds some spot that's easier to imagine as dark, less bright, or cloudy, or finds himself not wanting to look at a particular area, he *might* find his mind saying things like "I don't want to do this," "I can't do this," or even "I've *never* been able to visualize." If the patient finds an area that evokes these types of responses, I ask him to imagine the area is even darker, maybe even invisible. This may help him focus more easily on the area.

The area may be not merely dark, it might be a bit bizarre. I've had patients describe the dissociated part of the body with words like "decayed" and "confused." One patient said one side of the body was a rotten, stinking wharf, even though the other side of the body was filled with "normal" bright light.

If there is any darkness in a certain area, even splotchy or spotty darkness, cloudiness, or simply "something bizarre," then the person is very likely dissociated from that area of his body, or is on pause.

If any area inside the body is *easier* to imagine as being dark instead of light, and if that dark area is "heavy," "not moving," "weird" or "rotten," if it seems oppressively *motionless*, as if tied down or dead, that body part is probably dissociated away from normal consciousness.

Focusing on the negative

Right about now, you might be saying to yourself, "Focus on the dark? Focus on the *bad* stuff? That can't be good, that can't be *right…*"

Some people are surprised and then hesitant when I ask them to focus on dark or invisible places, what you might call "negative" images of their own body.

The need for some people to *focus on* and *pay attention to* the problem was one of the final breakthroughs in my Parkinson's research. People who had never been able to get lasting benefits from repeated attempts at "fill yourself with sweetness and light," or "positive thinking" suddenly found themselves able to get focused on and *permanently* remove their mental blocks.

As for the negative, dark images that some people see, they might show cultural influences. A patient who saw his injured leg only dimly, through "creepy stained glass" was raised in a Protestant faith. A patient who had grown up in Vietnam saw the classic, southeast-Asian Green Ghosts in her arm.

The images are in your mind, not your body

You can't *actually* see what's going on in your body with your mind's eye. Trying to visualize light or dark is merely an exercise in seeing what your mind is willing to consider. This exercise with light and dark is a way to diagnose the *mind*. It doesn't actually help diagnose the body.

Some patients have found it helpful to think of dissociation as causing a moat or barrier to be built around the brain cells associated with some body part or some aspect of a trauma memory.

"Neuron" is the name for a nerve cell in the brain. "Neural" means "having to do with neurons." When you tell yourself that you don't want to feel the pain or remember the trauma to your *foot*, for example, it's as if the brain builds a neural detour around the foot-awareness part of your brain. Subsequently, when you try to imagine light in your foot, you won't be able to. *Not* because the foot is injured, but because your mind is telling you, "There is no foot." Just as you instructed it.

The brain is obedient. If you tell it to lie or be in denial, it will lie or be in denial.

Also, *if* while doing the visualization exercises, *you* aren't the one doing the looking around inside, if you are instead employing some mentally produced minion or alter-ego to do the looking for you, you have probably dissociated from some body part, or maybe from your entire body. If a body part is easier to imagine as "*not* bright and perfect" or easier to imagine being in some location other than the location where the physical part actually is, such as sitting in a chair across the room from you, then dissociation is very likely going on.

Case study: fourth finger on the chopping block

I was working with a patient who had lost the use of her fourth finger ever since an accident with a kitchen knife cut the finger nearly to the bone. The finger appeared to be completely healed, but she couldn't feel or bend her finger. She was a professional pianist. She assumed this loss of feeling and flexibility meant the end of her career. Her doctor wrote off her loss as a permanent disability, explaining that cut nerves can't heal. (He was wrong. They can.)

I asked her to close her eyes and imagine she was looking inside her nose, then a healthy finger, and then her injured fourth finger. Not only was her fourth finger dark and motionless, she said it was impossible to find. It wasn't really there. Then I asked her to imagine she *did* have a fourth finger *somewhere*, and it was filled with beautiful light. She told me when she was able to do this. I asked her *where* the finger she was looking at was located.

She replied with surprise, "It's on the cutting board in my mother-in-law's house!"

I asked her to open her eyes, then gently asked. "How can your finger possibly resume feeling and flexibility if it's still in your mother-in-law's house?"

She was surprised that her mind had played this trick on her. She was able to restore her finger "back to life" by doing the light and energy exercise in her dark, motionless, and distant finger from which she had dissociated.

She had *also* been using self-induced pause since she was a child, when she was physically abused and kept locked in a very small closet most of the day by her caregiver, a family relation. The abuse lasted from age two to age seven. It ended when her mother came home early one day and discovered the situation.

Already being on self-induced pause probably made it easier for her to *completely* dissociate from her injured finger and even "leave it behind" when it got hurt.

She had recently started working with me on turning off her self-induced pause when the subject of her numb finger arose.

The re-association work on her finger was quick and easy. It took one session. Recovering from pause took longer: nearly a year.

Because of being on pause, her whole body felt sort of numb. She observed herself as if outside of her body. But as for her cut finger, even when she imaged she was observing herself from outside herself, her *finger* wasn't a part of her body. Her finger was in her mother-in-law's house.

The co-existence of both dissocation and pause is not unusual, and will be discussed in greater detail, in the next appendix.

Resistance to the very idea of a mental component

Many of my patients have *not* wanted to think that they have dissociated from some body part or are using self-induced dissociation or pause. Some have told me they preferred to have an incurable illness for "no reason at all" rather than consider the possibility that their own mind is playing a role in their sickness. One patient told me, "It's perfectly respectable to have Parkinson's disease. It's not respectable to have a mental problem."

For historical reasons that I'm not going to go deeply into here, western culture has long considered mentally-triggered health problems to be less "real" than physical ones, and even somewhat shameful, as if mind-activated problems indicate a lack of high morals.

If you're interested in when and how this attitude developed, please look up the details on René Descartes vs. the Pope on the mid-seventeenth century legal decision on the question of physical versus "spiritual" (including mental) illness. The conclusion of the legal debate was that, at risk of ex-communication, doctors agreed that they would study and care for the physical body, but that *all* mental/emotional issues would be considered spiritual problems and as such would belong to the realm of the church.

Thus, mental issues became *legally* separated from medical study. The results of this decision linger, still influencing western belief in the separation of physical and mental health. In eastern medicine, no such separation exists.

The fact is, nearly all illnesses have a mental component. Even the *rate* of healing from an injury or illness can be influenced by mental behaviors. The degree to which a person is physically sickened by physical and/or emotional damage or stress depends to a large extent on mental behaviors, including learned attitudes, that might seem completely unrelated.

As mentioned earlier, not every person chooses dissociation in response to trauma. But please don't think less of yourself if it turns out that you have dissociated from some problem or body part. It is a perfectly human thing to do. Dissociating is *not* an indication of a poor moral compass. It *may* be an indication of a relatively high intelligence and/or a high degree of mental self-control. It may be a *misguided* intelligence, driven by fear-based commands rather than wisdom, but a strong intelligence, nevertheless.

Then again, if you find yourself wanting to *justify* and continue clinging to the darkness that you have created inside yourself, it may be helpful to note that *some* people – people who are *not* using dissociation - can imagine bright light even in terribly injured or smashed-up parts of their bodies, even if they are in a significant deal of pain. Some might even automatically imagine angels getting in there and healing the injury. In fact, imagining light or miniature loved ones in a painful area is one of the more effective ways to reduce the pain and accelerate healing in any type of injury – slight or severe.

How one responds to pain or damage depends on one's personal style in dealing with difficulties. You *can* say that dissociation is not unusual. You cannot say that *everyone* does it, or that it's always automatic. Very often it's a decision.[1]

If, when visualizing an area inside the body, there is no light in an injured or sick area *and* the darkness is heavy, motionless, or invisible, it means the brain is trying to avoid acknowledging the existence of that area. This may be from automatic dissociation *or* from a mental command to yourself to "have no pain at that place" (self-induced dissociation).

---

[1] I highly recommend *Where There is Light*, an extraordinary memoir by Jacques Lusseyran. He was part of the French resistance during World War II. He was betrayed and captured. When he was dying in a Nazi concentration camp, he decided to once again fill himself with light, a practice he started when he permanently lost his eyesight as a young lad, a practice that he only abandoned when he was taken prisoner.

Once again filled with light, he recovered from his almost-fatal illness and fever. He survived the war even though most of his compatriots in the camp did not. His autobiographical book makes a profound argument against the negative practice of dissociation and the positive practice of literally keeping oneself filled with light regardless of circumstances.

A movie, *All the Light We Cannot See*, was released in 2015. The movie was based on a novel that was based on the memoir. I have no idea if the movie or novel gets the original author's message across. The actual autobiography was profoundly inspirational.

Either way, if a person is dissociated from an injury or trauma, there is no way that efficient, complete healing is going to occur until he mentally re-associates with the area in question.

Over time, if not re-associated, the "missing" body part and/or the area around it may become weak, or a source of chronic problems.

Case study: denial of dissociation from the gut

As already mentioned, many people do *not* want to even consider the *possibility* that they have dissociated from some body part. Patients sometimes *vigorously* resist the idea that they have dissociated from some part of their body.

For example, I sent an email to a long-distance patient with severe bowel disease asking him to assess if he might be dissociated from his intestines. I wrote to him about visualizing light inside, and also sent him some material on dissociation and pause.

He wrote back to me (I paraphrase), "I can dissociate at will, but I usually re-experience the trauma later, when it's safe. For example, I was attacked on the street one night, and I didn't cry until later. But I don't think I *store* trauma.

"I *might* have some degree of injury-based dissociation due to the extreme pain I have experienced in my gut, but my experience of life is not dissociated."

He continued, "It is easier for me to imagine my gut being dark, but I *can* send light through it if I really concentrate. When I imagine my gut, I imagine it *not* in the first person (it's not *me* seeing it). It's as if the gut has a "tiny me" that's sitting inside of my colon, or seeing my colon as though looking at a diagram. However, imagining that I'm looking at it directly, as if it's me on the inside of my body, looking out, is hard when I come to that specific part of my body.

"But I can do it eventually, I *can* send light there from me. Just not easily. Also, it looks like patchwork in there. Some light goes through, but there are some patches that are dark. Maybe those areas are injured or scarred. My problems with my gut started a couple of weeks after a very painful breakup with my long-time partner. But I don't think I'm dissociated from it. I can definitely *feel* pain in my gut. When I visualize the gut and see darkness, it's dark because it's *injured*, not because I'm dissociated."

The person quoted above, like many people, assumed that the dark areas in his gut looked dark because he was actually looking at injured areas. He was not.

He was confident that he was not dissociated because he *could* see light in the area, *temporarily*, *if* he worked really hard at it. Or if some minion worked at it on his behalf. Also, since he could *justify* the darkness as being due to pain, injury or scarring, he was sure he was not dissociated: he thought he was just the opposite: highly aware of what a mess his gut truly is, and therefore *not* dissociated. He was wrong.

Again, the imagination does *not* see what is actually, physically going on deep inside the body. The relative darkness or light in an *imagined*, given body part might have *nothing* to do what is physically happening in that area.

The *mind*, not the health status or injured status of an area, determines whether or not a given body part is going to be easy to imagine and filled with light, or is dark, or a mishmash, or speckled with dark and light areas or, for that matter, illuminated by creepy stained glass windows.

The brain is not clever

Why doesn't dissociation from pain stop when the pain stops?

In general, the brain is not very bright. It does *not* necessarily work in your best interests. The brain is *extremely* obedient. It learns through habit. For better or for worse, it does what you tell it to do. It thinks what you tell it to think. And it does so over and over, until you actively change the status quo.

The brain forms neural (brain cell) connections in response to your instructions and habits. The more *often* you tell yourself to do or think something, the stronger, deeper and faster those particular brain connections become. The brain is *not* the fixed, unchangeable switchboard, established and unchangeable since birth, that we were taught about in the 1900s.

The brain changes constantly. It changes in response to changing instructions from *you* and the responses you *choose* to make to external events: your own thoughts, decisions, and behaviors. As mentioned earlier, the brain's ability to change is called neuroplasticity.

If you think the same things over and over, the brain effectively becomes more rigid, more locked in to doing the same thing over and over. Still, no matter how locked in a person is, he *can* change his thoughts. It requires self-aware observation of one's thoughts and the replacement of outmoded or unwanted thoughts with the new, preferred thoughts.

If one of your instructions to the brain is "pretend the problem never happened," you will have to live with the consequences of that suppression until such time as you rescind your instructions.

Parkinson's disease from basic dissociation

As mentioned in chapter three, only about five percent of my Parkinson's patients inadvertently set in motion the electrical currents that create the symptoms of Parkinson's by using dissociation, not pause. Of that five percent, *most* of them were using *self-induced* dissociation.

However, a *very* few patients were using *basic*, *automatic* dissociation, after having gotten stuck in it following some trauma many years earlier.

Case study demonstrating basic dissociation

In the free Parkinson's clinic (1997 to 2003) at Five Branches, the acupuncture college where I teach, we had one Parkinson's patient who, during World War II, had dissociated from an entire day, the day he received his foot injury. The injury occurred just before an attack during which every man in his platoon died except him.

He *did* know he'd served in the war, but since the war he'd lived with *no* memories of that particular day.

Fifty years later, after receiving around six FSR sessions on the displaced bones in his foot, he announced during his session, "I just remembered an injury to that foot. I dropped an ammunition box on my foot. It was during the war. Pacific theater of operations." And then he dropped off to sleep.

A week later, during his next session, while his foot was being firmly held, he suddenly went into shock. He turned greenish, became nauseous, shook violently, and ran out of the building. He phoned several days later to explain that, up until that moment, he'd never remembered the day that "everyone died but me."

178

He'd never talked about it, never mentioned it to his wife. It was as if that day, for him, never existed.

Upon re-associating with the injury and then with that incomprehensible day, he became terrified, frantic. Even his sleep was traumatic. Every night after his re-association he had horrible nightmares of the scenes of carnage. He'd wake up screaming.

After his traumatic re-association, he refused to come in for further treatment. He announced, understandably, "I wish I had never been treated. I would rather have Parkinson's than have to live the rest of my life with these memories.

He ended up using very high doses of antiparkinson's medications to blunt his negative memories. The drugs helped him feel safe and even excessively ebullient in spite of his drug's side effects, which included violent, painful dyskinesia (muscle spasming).

The free clinic patients were treated in a big open room with no partitions. They, and very often their spouses, chatted amongst themselves before and during the treatments. A week prior to his violent re-association, his wife had confided to me, "He's not like your other Parkinson's patients. They're all so, I dunno, so *intense*, so *educated* or something. "

She went on, "He's just a regular Joe. He loves hanging out. He's never happier than when he has the barbeque spatula in one hand and a beer in the other."

She had been able to recognize, quickly, that he didn't have the classic Parkinson's personality characteristics that all the other patients in the group had: intensely focused, extremely intelligent, highly analytical, wary, and very word-based, or "left-brained."

He was different: he wasn't using self-induced pause, which in my experience is what *most* people with Parkinson's use. The use of self-induced pause is what creates what is medically known as the "Parkinson's personality." A person who is *not* using self-induced pause will probably *not* have this personality. In a group of people with Parkinson's, he may feel like he doesn't fit in.

This patient was only stuck on basic, *automatic* dissociation. He'd been in an emergency and had never gotten to a safe place to revisit it and turn off the dissociation…until he came to our clinic and received FSR treatment for his foot injury. That turned out to be his "safe place," a place safe enough to remember the horrendous events in his past. [1]

---

[1] In a weekend Yin Tui Na workshop in England, another person with Parkinson's said something similar about not being like the other Parkinson's patients. The workshop started with half an hour of introductory talk from me and a questions and answers session. Then we went around the half-circle of chairs, introducing ourselves. The next to last person was a thirty-five year old who'd been diagnosed with PD a few years earlier by a neurology "consultant" (what we call a "specialist" in the US).

After telling us her name, she said, "I don't belong here! I'm not like you people."

As it turns out, she was correct. She had injured her arm flipping a fry basket at the fish shop where she worked. The next day, her arm could barely move. It certainly didn't "swing" when she walked. Her shoulder joint, painful and seriously displaced, tremored when she tried to use it.

She had no other symptoms of Parkinson's. Her doctor had *egregiously* misdiagnosed her painful shoulder and unusable arm as Parkinson's based on two symptoms: her shaky arm, which he diagnosed as "tremor," and "lack of arm swing while walking."

During the lunch break, I did Yin Tui Na on her grossly displaced arm/shoulder joint. After her upper arm popped back into the shoulder socket, she *immediately* had normal use of her arm, an arm swing, and her tremor was completely gone, for good. The pain was gone. She had been *horribly*

Case study: arm in the coffin pose

For another example of dissociation, I had a patient in her early thirties with very early symptoms of Parkinson's, including a bit of right-side foot shuffling, mildly reduced right-side arm swing, a pushed-forward neck / head, and an intermittent tremor that was very slowly increasing in frequency.

When asked to imagine light in her tremory arm, she replied, "That's funny...my actual arm is lying by my side, and it's dark. But when I imagine it being full of light, *that* arm is lying across my chest, like how you put someone's arms in a coffin. Well..." she continued, "*that* can't be helping the situation! No wonder that arm tremors!" She laughed out loud.

She thought this mental illusion was really funny, which is *not* typical of the Parkinson's personality. She quickly mentally integrated her "coffin arm" with her actual arm and thought nothing of it.

It turns out, she had broken that arm when she was four years old.

She recovered very quickly, over the course of two months, from her Parkinson's symptoms and from an assortment of the recovery symptoms. She had been merely dissociated from her arm. She was *not* on pause.

She also did not have the Parkinson's personality, which is most often related to self-induced pause: wariness; feeling apart from others; unable to understand that phrases like "open your heart" and "speak from your heart" are *literal*, not metaphorical.

She was a professional musician, one of several of my professional-musician patients with Parkinson's who were merely dissociated and were *not* stuck on pause.

She was merely dissociated from her arm. She did not have any of the other personality and comprehension behaviors that are discussed in the book *Recovery from Parkinson's*. That book is available for free download at www.pdrecovery.org, or in hard copy at JaniceHadlock.com.

In my few patients with Parkinson's who only had *basic* dissociation, such as the man described above who'd dropped an ammunition box on his foot the day all his fellow soldiers died, and the woman with her dissociated arm resting in the "coffin" pose, they usually needed only a few treatment sessions of FSR until their Parkinson's symptoms evaporated.

---

misdiagnosed. The drugs she'd been taking for three years had never helped, and she had side effects from them and was addicted to them.

But, she had *never* had Parkinson's. More to the point, after a *very* short time in a room full of people with PD, it had been obvious to her that she was in a room full of people who were "different" from her.

She was a very sweet, easy-going woman, a high school dropout who worked in a fry shop. She had immediately felt that everyone else in the room was articulate and analytical [not her words], an independent thinker, and friendly enough but highly alert and with what you might call an "edge." These are all characteristics of self-induced pause.

She felt very much out of place, even "in over her head," in the company of people who actually had Parkinson's, all of them due to self-induced pause. And she was right. She really did *not* fit in. She had *never* had Parkinson's disease.

They didn't need to "cauterize" brain cells or "destroy" the brain cells of a wrong mental habit, as described in chapter six.

Unlike these few examples, *most* people with Parkinson's (in my experience) who are not on pause but who *have* dissociated had the *self-induced* type of dissociation: during their FSR sessions, they remembered giving themselves instructions to ignore or "not have" an injured body part.

As noted earlier, about five percent of my hundreds of patients with Parkinson's have had a dissociation situation in place, *not* a pause situation.

Dissociation summary

People with either basic dissociation or self-induced dissociation will see their "dark" areas as *immobile*, *heavy*, *lifeless* or even *"non-existent."* If imagined as being filled with light, the body part in question might appear in a different location from the actual body part. If *mentally* forced to be reluctantly filled with light, the body part might even be perceived as being viewed by someone or something other than oneself.

If a person is dissociated, he should first use the "light and energy" technique in this book in chapter five.

If, after using this technique, the dark area returns, shape shifts, or moves evasively, the person probably has self-induced dissociation and should next use the techniques in this book in chapter six.

As noted earlier, people can be using both dissociation and pause. Sometimes, terminating one of these two conditions will reveal that the other condition is present.

Treat whichever condition is presenting at the moment, whichever is dominant at the moment.

Appendix II

Diagnosing pause

Diagnosing pause: method #1 Dark and agitated

You will recall from the previous appendix that an area that your mind perceives as dark and immobile is an area from which you've dissociated. Finding an area that your mind perceives as dark and vibrating, or agitated in any way, suggests that you are stuck on pause.

It's time for a lengthier discussion of just what is meant by "agitated or vibrating."

"Agitation"

Whether you've found one dark place or a few dark places, or your whole body is dark and yet you've homed in a very dark*est* or *most* non-existent places in your body, the next thing you're going to notice is if this area is moving, or not.

Gaze at the dark area. Notice if there is an oppressive heaviness, a stillness, an immobility in the darkest part of the dark area. You will recall from the previous chapter that *this* behavior suggests dissociation.

However, if this area is agitated or moving in *any* way, it suggests that this part of your body, or more likely your whole body, is using pause.

When I say "agitated," I mean *any* type of movement. The area may appear as if the atoms are moving about too quickly. Or as if the microscopic bits, the capillaries or the cell walls, are moving. The area might appear to be rippling, or have waves of "smoke" traveling through. There might be tiny, purely imaginary quaking, or tremoring. The area might seem sludgy, twitching, or even "bubbling."

It doesn't matter exactly what *kind* of "movement" behavior is being exhibited, or where. If your brain is perceiving some part of you as exhibiting this behavior, your brain is also behaving, to some degree, as if you are in profound, near-death shock: on pause.

Most people will see this agitation in the area that was injured. However, some people may also see some type of "dark and agitated" behavior at the sacrum (the bone at the base of the spine), the seventh cervical vertebra (at the base of the neck, near the shoulders), around the heart, or in a few cases, throughout the entire body.

The injury area *and* some other dark area might *both* be agitated.

Deciding whether or not the area is agitated or motionless should only take about five to ten seconds. Thirty seconds, tops.

The body part in question will probably *not* be exhibiting any physical movement or tremoring that's visible to an outside observer. A person with essential tremor or Parkinson's tremor will not necessary be *visibly* tremoring in the same parts of the body that are perceived as agitated *internally*, in the dark place(s). For example, a person with a hand tremor will not usually visualize an internally dark and agitated hand, but he might visualize a dark and agitated place in the neck.

The imagined, *visualized* agitation shows how your *brain* is perceiving this area. The brain is telling you it perceives the area as agitated and/or moving in some way, shape, or form. This brain perception of movement or agitation, whether large or subtle, occurs because the body part in question is trying to get your brain's attention so that it can ask the crucial question: "Is it OK to come back to life? Is the danger gone? Is the predator gone?"

This is very different from dissociation. In dissociation, the brain is pretending that the body part doesn't exist. Therefore, when you try to imagine this body part, nothing moves. The area might be motionless or "heavy" or might not even exist.

But if you are dealing with an unresolved trauma or shock, your physical body is *actively trying* to get your brain's attention. It wants to get your brain's attention because *only* the brain can determine if the situation is now safe enough that pause can be turned off.

That's why mentally gazing at a part of your body that is stuck on pause will present as if this very dark, medium dark, smoky, or slightly dim area is agitated or moving in some way.

As an aside, a normal part in coming out of shock or full-body anesthesia is the subtle or obvious *physical* shaking or tremoring, usually occurs body-wide. This perfectly natural tremoring is supposed to get the brain's attention so that the brain can assess the situation and come out of pause as soon as it is safe to do so.

BUT, so long as the brain says, "We might still be at risk" or "Only an idiot could ever think he's safe," pause will not be turned off. Subtle, internal agitation, or not-so-subtle agitation in the case of palpable, visible tremor, will continue, but it will also continue to be ignored by the brain because the brain has determined that "it's not safe yet."

The reason the body part that's perceived as being agitated needs to get agreement from the brain is this: the body part does not have enough information to decide if things are now safe. The brain has connections to the eyes, ears, skin, and a sense of smell. The brain has the ability to assess. Therefore, the brain, not the body part, has the authority to decide whether or not a life-threatening risk is still present.

The vibrating, tremoring, or even "bubbling" or "burning" that is perceived in some traumatized body part that is imagined as dark or even somewhat dim can be thought of as the traumatized area "waving its hands" at the brain, trying to get the brain's attention so that the process of coming out of pause can be initiated. The area is perceived as somewhat dark or dim because the brain, in these cases, is trying to ignore that area's constant call for recognition and the question as to whether or not it's safe yet.

The agitation signal will continue to be given off by the body part(s) that are stuck on pause until the brain decides that the situation *is* now safe enough and calls the all clear.

More than one process at work

If you going to self-diagnose which type of mental-diversion process, if any, you're using, please be aware that you might be using more than one. *Not* everyone limits himself to just one type or another. People don't necessary have *only* dissociation, self-induced dissociation, pause, or self-induced pause.

Many people use *more* than one of the above techniques for avoiding physical or emotional pain. For example, in the previous appendix, the person with a "missing" fourth finger was using both dissociation and pause.

I'm being painfully redundant about this because people who are using self-induced pause tend to get very anxious about making sure they are making the "correct" diagnosis. Please, don't be so exacting, because what you are looking for might be a moving target. If, like most people with Parkinson's, you are using self-induced pause, you may well be using *several* pain avoidance techniques. If this is the case, in the big picture, whether or not you recover from your health problems won't depend on getting your diagnosis "exactly right." If you are using self-induced pause, recovering from your health problems might mostly depend on learning how to be a bit more easy going, feeling safe no matter what, and trusting your heart to guide you to what you need. The opposite of being "exactly right."

As for what "exactly" is going on in your mind in terms of dissociation *versus* pause, you might actually be using both.

We can all create our own rules in our own brain as to how we are going to stay away from things we don't like. Each person can combine and layer his reality-hiding mental behaviors in any way he likes. The main thing to keep in mind is that, prior to receiving any FSR treatment, any pause-related behaviors should be treated first, if they exist. After pause is *permanently* turned off (meaning it doesn't show up again an hour or a few days later), then dissociation behaviors can be addressed. If pause and dissociation both exist and are layered, treat whatever is presenting at the moment.

The following non-Parkinson's case study might help make this point.

Case study: broken bones and head injury on the golf course

A patient, female, age 72, a healthy, very busy professional and a lifetime golfer had burning pain in her legs. The pain was much worse in the evenings, or whenever she was pressed for time or under stress.

A year earlier, a golf cart had rolled over and landed on her right foot, ankle, and lower leg, breaking several bones in her foot. The event had also thrown her onto her head.

She had worn a heavy stabilizing boot for a few weeks, but decided it was an inconvenience and stopped wearing it. Instead, she told herself, "I don't need this. I'm not going to let this slow me down!" (She didn't remember having given herself these instructions until *after* she did the techniques for turning off self-induced dissociation.)

From that moment, she had no pain in her foot and was able to move normally. She had the usual follow-up visit with her doctor after six weeks. The doctor was concerned about how the foot moved. She x-rayed the foot and found that the bones were still broken.

Even so, my patient refused to resume wearing the therapeutic "boot." She assumed that the bones would heal, given time, considering that she no longer had any pain.

About six months later, the burning pain in the legs showed up. At the time, she associated it with an allergic rash that she got while using a soy-based probiotic (gut bacteria supplement). When she stopped using the probiotic, the rash on her chest cleared up, but the heat in her legs remained. By the time she came to see me, the heat in her legs was becoming extreme, and in the evenings or during stress, it was nearly unbearable.

When I started working with her, it was clear that the bones were still slightly displaced and very possibly still broken.

I did Yin Tui Na on the lower leg, ankle, and foot, but *first*, I had her visually imagine a quick scan of various areas in her body, including all the areas that she knew had been injured.

The back of her skull was dark and heavy, not moving, as were her right shoulder, the medial (inner) side of her right knee, and her lateral (outer) right ankle.

When she imagined looking at her third cervical vertebra (neck bone), about an inch down from the base of the skull, she saw an area that was dark and vibrating. She saw another area that was dark and "burning" (which qualifies as vibrating or agitated) just below her right knee on the lateral side, and another on her right ankle on the medial side.

She had a collection of locations with either self-induced dissociation and/or pause. The areas that were dark and agitated were locations where her injuries had been dangerous enough that, on some level of consciousness she had evidentially felt she was at genuine risk of death – and had subsequently failed to deal with the trauma.

The areas that were dark and not moving had obviously been injured, but she had been able to successfully command herself to dissociate from them ("I don't need this!")

In my office, she re-connected with the dissociated areas using the technique in chapter five for basic dissociation. She turned off pause in the body parts that were dark and vibrating by using the five steps that turn off basic pause.

I treated her foot with Yin Tui Na. Bones slid back into place, the muscles in her leg relaxed.

She had no heat symptoms for the next twenty-four hours. But the symptoms returned the next evening, in response to thinking about an upcoming golf event.

At our next session, when she told me her symptoms returned after being gone for a while, I said I suspected she was dealing with a self-induced situation. She did not agree. She had not yet remembered her own instructions: "I don't need this! I refuse to feel this pain."

So once again, in the dark areas I had her do the light and energy exercise in chapter five. In the agitated areas, I had her go through the steps that turn off pause.

Even though the invisible friend she invoked to help her feel safe enough to turn off pause *assured* her she was not at risk of imminent death (death in the next few minutes) from the golf cart injury, she had a hard time agreeing with him (steps two and three, described in chapter one of *Stuck on Pause*).

As in our previous session, she had a bit of a struggle with the pause exercise, going back and forth between what her friend was cheerful confirming: "You're *not* at risk of imminent death!" and what *she* wanted to say: "But I *am* at risk of imminent death!" She battled this out for about two minutes – which seems like a long time if you're in the middle of it.

She finally said to me, out loud, that she was *not* at risk of imminent death from the golf cart injury. It was hard for her to get those words out.

She immediately took a deep breath and was able to do the neck bobble and shiver that occurs when pause is turned off.

Her legs had no heat for nearly a week.

However, after six days with no burning heat in her legs, she set up a golf date for the next day. The burning pain in her legs returned that night, full bore. It was gone in the morning, but resumed for the whole time she was on the golf course.

Since her symptoms had been gone for six days, her problem was obviously no longer the broken bones or being stuck on basic dissociation or pause. She was obviously in a *self-induced* condition. When I saw her next, she was once again using a combination of pause behaviors (visualizing body parts as dark and agitated) and dissociation behaviors (dark and immobilized) in areas that had previously been "cleaned up."

At this point, she laughingly admitted that her subconscious was playing tricks on her.

This time, I led her through the treatment for *self-induced* dissociation in her injured areas, the exercises in chapter six of this book.

Following this, the *new* darkest area was at the base of the spine: in the sacrum, an area that is often dark and agitated or vibrating when a person is in a near-death condition. In her case, it was dark and immobile, not dark and vibrating. Therefore, she and I could conclude that she had dissociated from this area.

She did the technique in chapter five for re-associating. After this, she could see that the sacrum was *now* dark and *vibrating* – which is typical for a severe, shock-inducing injury.

After clearing up the *pause* behavior in the sacrum, which had previously been masked by the *dissociation* behavior in the sacrum, she had no more episodes of burning pain in her legs.

As mentioned earlier, brain behaviors can build layers of self-protection mechanisms around a given area. Treat whatever is presenting at the time. If, after treatment, another type of situation appears, then treat that type of situation.

She told me later, she hadn't even realized it consciously, but for six months she had been subconsciously avoiding the golf course and even finding ways to get out of golf dates. After getting rid of her self-induced dissociation *and* pause, in various locations, she once again found herself keenly looking forward to getting out on the links.

This above case study shows how the patient was diagnosed, at first, with *both* pause *and* dissociation. At first, she vehemently did *not* agree that she might also have created some self-induced behaviors. She was highly intelligent and felt that she would never do anything psychologically "wrong" in her own mind.

However, after her symptoms and her imagined dark areas resolved in the short term but kept returning over time, she was reluctantly able to admit that her mind seemed to be contributing to her problem. After she started doing techniques in chapter six for getting rid of her own, self-created brain instructions, she healed quickly and normally. This case study beautifully demonstrates how both dissociation and pause can co-exist, even in response to a single event.

Diagnosing pause: method #2   Moving the energy, or not

You can start by comparing what it feels like to *be* on pause and to *not* be on pause. If you are *not* already stuck on pause, you can temporarily experience and compare these two states by doing the following exercises. If you suspect you *are* stuck on pause these exercises might help you confirm or deny your diagnosis.

1) *Not* on pause:

Close your eyes. Imagine a current moving up your back, from the lowest part of the back, either your coccyx or sacrum, up into the neck and head. The current is about an eighth of an inch under the skin and about a quarter of an inch wide. In Chinese medicine, this is called the "Du" channel.

Your imaginary current can be made out of anything moveable: light, electricity, wind, water, warmth, or a tingly feeling – anything at all that you can imagine as moving.

Pretend you can feel this energy as it flows just under the skin that lies over the spine, from the base of the spine, up the neck and *into* the head, then through the midbrain over to the forehead, where it emerges from the head and flows down to the upper lip and into the mouth.

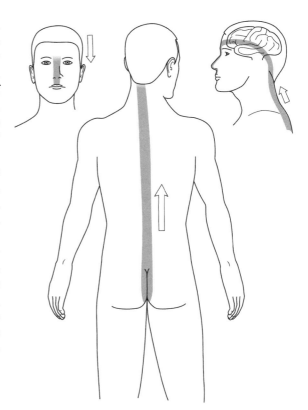

Fig. Appx II. 1   The Du channel when awake

If your immediate response to these instructions was "I can't do visualization," or if this exercise is difficult, you may well be on pause.

If you *can* easily imagine a current moving up into the neck and head and if it feels good, normal, and even automatic, requiring no mental labor, then you are probably not stuck on pause.

2) On pause:

After doing the previous exercise with the Du channel flowing up into the neck and head, now *stop* the flow of the Du channel at the base of the neck. Do *not* allow any current to flow up into the head. Feel that you have created a holding pattern, a standing wave, in the current of energy that runs just under your skin, directly over your spine. There might be energy there, but it's *not* moving into the neck or head. Don't let any energy flow into your neck and head from your Du channel.

In the ancient Chinese description, when this stoppage occurs, the Du channel has ceased to be a river, and has become like a "reservoir."

Note: the drawing of the Du channel on pause has *no* arrows showing directional movement.

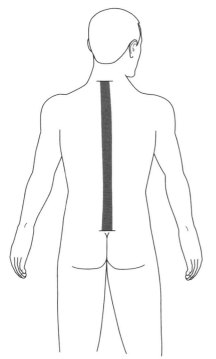

Maintain this holding pattern for up to five inutes, if you can stand to do it for that long.

After about five minutes or maybe even start noticing the changes in your muscles, :ial expression, your thoughts, and your ability oy in your heart.

Your muscles may feel as if they are tensing t. Your arms might even be bending at the pulling in, tightening up. Your facial muscles :el heavy.

Your facial expression might be getting stony. houghts may be wary, and might include such as "I really don't like this" or even "This ble; I feel like I'm dying." Your sense of a resonant area in your heart that expands or s with joy or fear, respectively, will feel leadened.

Fig Appx II.2   The Du channel on pause

After a bit longer, still maintaining this holding pattern, you might perceive yourself as being slightly "outside" of your own body. A common "outside" location is a quarter inch or so behind the back of the neck. These are all symptoms of being on pause.

Done? Be *sure* to let the current resume moving through your head again.

Don't worry about getting stuck in this mode. As soon as you resume the flow of energy through your head, all those weird pause symptoms will go away...assuming you were *not* already stuck on pause before you started this exercise. If you were already on pause, you won't feel much difference, if any, while doing the healthy and the pause parts of the exercise.

Assessment

If doing the second exercise made you feel really weird, or at least somehow different from how you usually feel, then you are not normally using pause mode. By the way, the way you felt while doing the exercise is what it feels like to have early-stage pause-based idiopathic Parkinson's disease.

If you feel more "normal" or more "natural" or it's "easier" when you are *preventing* current from going into your head or you feel more familiar with *allowing* the current to stop at the base of the skull, then you are probably stuck on pause.

If current moving through up your neck and into your head in the first part of this exercise made you feel a little giddy at first (an unaccustomed surge of dopamine release that won't last), *or* even *more* wary than usual or more vulnerable, or maybe experiencing the thought, "I shouldn't be doing this" or, if you feel a tightening or discomfort, or even the fear of *potential* discomfort, in your heart, stomach, throat or other area, if you simply felt "not normal," "not safe," or if you simply could not do it, couldn't feel anything, or didn't understand the assignment, you are very likely stuck on pause.

For that matter, if you do not know what is *meant* by the words "the resonant area in your heart that expands or contracts with joy or fear, respectively," you are probably stuck on pause and may have been for a long, long time. Ditto if the references to "heart feeling" and/or "heart resonance" (actual, somatic *sensations*) in this book don't mean anything to you in terms of experiencing actual sensation in the chest.

If you are accustomed to thinking that phrases such as "open your heart" or "feel in your heart" mean "think good thoughts" or "be nice" as opposed to what they actually mean, you may be stuck on pause. These phrases are actually exhortations to redirect more of your awareness towards the actual *sensations* of resonance-driven changes in the electrical patterns in the pericardium (the highly conductive connective tissue around the heart) and thus feel more connected to things outside of yourself.

Lack of Du channel flow is not *always* pause

If you have a very hard time imagining a specific part of the Du channel, or if the energy in the Du channel seems to move in fits and starts or is difficult to even imagine, you *might* have electrical currents stuck on pause **or** there may be an unhealed back, neck, skull, or brain injury, with basic dissociation or pause from the injury.

If you are aware of a history of spine, neck, or head injury, I highly recommend a light touch cranio-sacral treatment or two to either turn off basic dissociation or pause or maybe rule them out. Many times a person with a history of concussion or spinal injury has come to me with symptoms that are similar to pause, but the only treatment needed was one or two cransio-sacral sessions.[1]

Often, a person who has displacements in the skull, neck, or spine due to injury will still be able to imagine light in those areas. In these cases, the person might not have dissociated from the problem, but might just need a little bit of steady, hands-on support so that his body can re-align itself back into its correct layout.

But if the person cannot even imagine his head, neck or spine being filled with light, he might be dealing with dissociation from these areas and/or a pause situation. How to tell which?

---

[1] Many massage therapists are trained in light touch cranio-sacral therapy. (Not chiropractic cranio-sacral therapy, which can be, in some cases, a completely different type of treatment.) If there is no one in your area who has trained in this modality, visit chapter fifteen in this book.

Motionless or agitated, again

How can you tell if dark, unmoving energy blocking the spine or the Du channel is caused by pause or is caused by a dissociated injury? The same way you assess a dark area anywhere in the body.

Look into the center of the dark area, or the darkest part of the area that seems blocked.

If it is easier to imagine this area is dark instead of light *and* if it's easier to imagine it's dark and *heavy*, like an inanimate, *unmoving* lump, you've probably dissociated from an injury in that area, thus preventing healing of the injury.

If it's easier to imagine that the area is dark instead of light *but* subtle agitation or quivering is occurring, you are probably stuck on pause from an injury in this area.

If the dark area is microscopically trembling or vibrating, the area might be the *site* of a near-death shock/injury that has put you on pause. In addition to "faintly trembling" or "as if the atoms are vibrating," people on pause variously have described their imagined movement at their dark areas as bubbling, burning, tremulous, and even sludgy or sticky.

It doesn't matter *how* it's moving. Just decide if the darkest part of the dark area seems to be motionless or non-existent (dissociation) or if it is somehow agitated or moving strangely (pause).

Then again, if the area seems to moving in a pleasant, back and forth manner, maybe even in time with your breathing, that's just normal. But *if* the area is easier to imagine as dark than light, it's unlikely that there will be "pleasant" movement going on.

If dissociated, and the dissociation was *not* self-induced, if it is just basic dissociation that has gotten stuck, then use the techniques in chapter five to turn it off.

If on pause, and pause mode was *not* self-induced, if it just basic pause that has gotten stuck, then going through the five steps for turning off basic pause (in chapter one of the book *Stuck on Pause*) while focused on this specific area might well turn off pause.

Diagnosing pause #3: Inside the body or outside the body

Another test for whether or not you are on pause is determining if you are going through your moments of self-awareness by *feeling* your body from the inside *or* by imagining you are *looking* at yourself from some location outside of your actual body.

If you tend to observe or think of your body as if you are outside of it, looking at yourself instead of *feeling* your existence by using the resonance of your heart (pericardium, actually) as your primary point of reference, you are very likely stuck on pause.

If, when you speak, you imagine the words appearing in front of you on the "video screen" of your imagination, you may be stuck on pause.

If you mentally use *words* to self-assess how you are feeling instead of checking in with your wordless heart-area *sensations* of expansion and contraction you may be stuck on pause.

If you have no idea what I mean by "*feeling* your body from the inside" or "heart sensations" you are probably stuck on pause. The term "heart sensations" does not refer to heart palpitations, which are the worrisome, tangible sensations of your heart's beating. My usage of the phrase "heart sensations" refers to the subtle sense of expansion and contraction in the chest, in the area *around* the heart, that can be felt (by most people) when experiencing something poignant or beautiful, or something dreadful, respectively.

The Inside or outside the body exercise

Close your eyes. Imagine you are walking down a lovely tree-lined street. It's a beautiful day. Birds are chirping. A gentle breeze is rustling the leaves. The sky is blue.

Take five to ten seconds to imagine this.

Are you *looking* at your body, or are you experiencing the stroll from *inside* your body, *feeling* your sensations of walking and feeling the expansion in your heart area as you hear the birds?

If you are outside of your body, *can* you imagine yourself inside your body, experiencing the sensations of stride from within?

If you are *unable* to imagine yourself inside your body, or it takes a bit of work, or it's hard to make your sensory awareness *stay* inside once it's put there, there is a very good chance you are on pause. If this is the case, the next step is to imagine looking around inside your body. Find the very darkest place. See if it is motionless or agitated.

Diagnosing pause #4:   Yoga and Qi Gong responses

If years of yoga, meditation, Qi Gong, Tai Ji (aka Tai Chi) have not brought you the promised heart feelings of peaceful, expansive joy, you may be on pause. If you have done years of the above practices and have done it without feeling increasing joy and energy flooding various the body parts as they are moved or are focused on, you may be on pause.

If you do the above types of movement while trying to make your movements symmetrical, or uniform, or "correct," you may well be on pause.

If you like doing the yogic "corpse pose" because it lets you "turn off" and/or pretend you are dead, you may be on pause.

On the other hand, *if* you enjoy doing these types of self-improvement exercises because they help you turn off your internal monologue and savor, *wordlessly*, the heightened awareness of somatic energy in your various body parts, you are probably *not* on pause.

If you like doing the yogic "corpse pose" because you love the heightened awareness of energy being released from your muscles and flowing up your spine and into your head and heart, and your increased awareness of somatic resonance in the deep stillness of your body, you are probably *not* on pause.

I have worked with hundreds of people who have Parkinson's disease. Most of them, around ninety-five percent, were stuck on self-induced pause. Nearly all of the ones who have steadily practiced the meditative arts (a significant percent) have told me that their decades of silent meditation, yoga asanas, or other "spiritual" movement exercises have *not* led to increased awareness of inner joy or heart resonance. Just the opposite: they have felt less and less joy and/or less heart awareness over the years, despite decades of doing these supposedly "uplifting" exercises.

Also, many of them have said that "corpse" is their favorite yoga pose. [1]

---

[1] Vocabulary note: for those who do certain types of Buddhist meditation, remember that going into the so-called "emptiness" refers to turning off ego-driven thoughts and constant mental chatter. It does *not* mean becoming *numb* to the joy that vibrates silently behind every atom. The use

Diagnosing pause #5:   How do you move?

If you move by mentally *commanding* your body to move rather than by enjoying the vibrant or languorous sensations of motor actions that occur automatically and immediately in response to thinking about or imagining moving your body, and especially if you don't know what this sentence means, you may well be stuck on pause.

Other easy things to look for

Unhealed injury, lipomas, moles that are slowly increasing in size, or even fungus intruding under the toenails or fingernails are a few examples of "not healing properly" situations in which the somewhat bizarre electrical patterns of pause, or maybe dissociation, *might* be preventing some location in the body from doing its normal job of healing from physical injuries, illnesses, or everyday wear and tear. Imagine looking around inside, in the locations of these types of problem areas.

Is it easier to imagine as dark? Is it dark and motionless? Dark and agitated?

Finally, a diagnostic reminder: a person who is stuck on pause doesn't necessarily *look* as if he is in shock. He needn't appear stunned or blank-faced. For years, maybe decades, he might have been able to stay highly mobile via commanding himself to use "emergency" thoughts, thus releasing neural norepinephrine (a relative of adrenaline). He might be able to instruct himself to be "socially correct," smiling and sincerely conforming to the rules of polite conduct. However, unlike people for whom these behaviors flow somewhat naturally, from the heart, the person who is running pause in the background will always be performing these behaviors somewhat self-consciously, using an adrenaline-like neural override and using, for the most part, brain-based logic and self-awareness even though he may be *talking* about spontaneity, heart and love.

This subject is discussed in great detail in *Stuck on Pause*.

---

of the word "emptiness" is a poor translation. "Love-filled absence of ego" might have been a better choice. I have had Buddhist patients, including Buddhist monks and even teachers, who were stuck on pause, who had Parkinson's disease. In every case, they had assumed that the word "emptiness" means numbness, even joylessness!

To illustrate the translation challenges, let me share a story about signage in India, the homeland of the Buddha. I noticed, in ashrams in India, dual language signs in Hindi and English at the entrance to some of the meditation halls. The Hindi message had two words. The first word is a verb that can mean "keep" or stay." (This same verb is used in signs that mean, "Keep off the grass," or you might say, "Stay off the grass.") The second word in the phrase is "shanti," which is usually translated into English as "peace." These two words together *might* be translated into English as "keep peaceful: full of quiet, radiant, joy."

But the sign's translation into English said, "Maintain silence."

The words shanti (peace) and silence have utterly different *underlying* meanings. Joy is implied in the first. Self-control and rigidity is implied in the second.

This is just to point out how hard it can be to put into English the words and phrases from other languages that have to do with heart-joy and peace.

Many English speakers who are stuck on pause even think that the word "peace" means "motionless," and point for an example to the phrase, "a peaceful evening." I doubt the word "motionless" could be applied to the greatly dynamic Jesus, who is sometimes described as a "Prince of Peace." Peace is a dynamic heart-feeling. Many people stuck on pause are not able to access this feeling, or even understand that the word peace can *refer* to an actual feeling.

"Everything's dark" or "There's nothing to see!"

I mentioned earlier that we would be getting around to the question about the whole body being imagined as dark. If you cannot imagine light anywhere in your body, not even in your nose or earlobes, don't be alarmed. You are not alone.

Try this: imagine that you *do* have a body somewhere that's filled with beautiful light, but it doesn't have to be *inside* of you.

Some patients have seen their beautiful light-filled body back at the lake, at a childhood summer camp. Others have seen it across the room, or hovering a few inches above their physical body.

Next, see how you feel about putting that beautiful body, full of light, back into your own physical body.

If it's easy to do and the body of light stays inside you and you can now visualize yourself easily as being full of light – and the light doesn't leave – then that's great. You might have gotten dissociated or stuck on pause during an injury and never turned it off. If your body is once again full of light and you notice increased awareness of sensation in your body, you may have successfully turned off the problem.

If *most* of your physical body can be filled with light but some limb, digits, or some other body part are outside of your physical body, you may be only dissociated from the body part that isn't where it should be. You might *not* be on pause. Check by looking to see if your brain perceives the area is dark and heavy or unmoving, *or* if it's dark and agitated or moving in any way.

If, as is common in Parkinson's, you can't put your "beautiful light body" into your actual physical body, or if it would feel "disgusting" to do so, or "wrong," or if any other negative emotion would result if your imagined body was inserted back into your physical body, you are probably using pause mode, and the odds are good that it is self-induced. Differentiating between basic pause and self-induced pause is discussed in the book *Stuck on Pause*.

If you imagine that your "body made of light" is not inside your actual body, it's no wonder that your actual body must be imagined as full of darkness. Fine. Don't worry. These are just behaviors of the imagination. You actually *are* alive and full of energy, even if your mind is resisting the idea.

Other places where agitation might occur

Even if you have found a dark area at the site of an old injury, you might want to mentally imagine looking at a few other places, as well.

If the original trauma was body-wide, such as near-drowning, a concussion, or anaphylactic shock, a dark vibrating area may well be located in the sacrum. If the trauma was concussion, a dark and vibrating place might be in the head but also at the base of the neck.

If the trauma was located at a specific body part, for example, the right knee or the left elbow, the area that is darkest and vibrating *might* be at the injury site. Or, at the sacrum. Or *both* the injury site and the sacrum. Or for that matter, it might be over the whole right side, or left side, of the body.

The more life-threatening the injury, or the more forcefully that pause was self-induced, the more likely it is, in my patients' experiences, that there will be some darkness and agitation in the sacrum, or the base of the neck, and/or the heart area. Even if there is agitation in some injury area(s), the sacrum, base of neck, or heart areas might *also* be involved.

Summary

Basic pause

If you do the pause-diagnosing exercises in this chapter and you find that some dark area(s) in your body are agitated or moving, you most likely are stuck on pause.

If you have basic pause, and you go through the steps involved in convincingly affirming that the situation is now safe enough, pause should automatically turn off: you'll take a deep, audible breath. Your head will wobble high on the neck, turning the vagus nerve back on. A frisson will run down your spine, turning the spinal nerves and the adrenal glands back on.

This is how *basic* pause gets turned off.

If you determine that you are stuck on pause, please read Stuck on Pause, available online for free download at www.pdrecovery.org or in hard copy (book form) at JaniceHadlock.com.

This book has very detailed, specific instructions that will enable you to turn off this _biological_ behavior.

Self-induced pause

Self-induced pause will *manifest* in the same way as basic pause: the dark areas or the entire dark body will seem to have some kind of agitation or movement going on. Energy won't travel easily from the spine into the head, and so on.

However, the underlying *cause* of self-induced pause is *completely* different from that of basic pause.

Self-induced pause occurs when a person has commanded himself to feel no pain, to rise above pain, to play dead, or some other body-wide instruction: commanded himself to play a role.

With self-induced pause, the brain has activated a personality that uses pause in order to *comply* with the instruction. The brain is not going to turn off pause until the person rescinds the command *or* during those moments when the brain decides that the command doesn't apply.

In a person who is stuck on self-induced pause, the problem is that the person never got around to turning off that instruction. The mental instruction, still working away as instructed, is what prevents pause from turning off. The instruction is what keeps the darkness and agitation in place.

A person with self-induced pause might do the techniques for turning off pause, and might even succeed in turning off pause several times an hour, but pause will keep re-establishing itself because the command to "feel no pain," "rise above fear," or "be in control of what you feel" is still working away.

If you are able to get rid of your on-pause behaviors, including turning off the visualized agitation or movement in some part of your body BUT the behavior returns within a few minutes, hours, or days, then you most likely have self-induced pause. If you can't permanently turn off pause because it keeps coming back, or if you don't *want* to turn off pause, then you are most likely using *self-induced* pause.

Not *wanting* to turn off pause is more common than you might think. Very emphatic remarks from many of my patients, remarks such as "Only an *idiot* would want to stop being afraid!" and "It's just *smart* to be anxious all the time!" show how deeply a person can come to associate being on pause with being intellectually and/or morally superior.

People making these types of remarks also tend to give little credibility to the idea that their inability to feel joyful expansion of their own hearts is diminishing their experience of life.

Oppositely, a common sentiment expressed by people who've *recovered* from Parkinson's is "Gee. I was such a fool. I wanted to recover from Parkinson's so I could go back to being the in-control person I'd been before. Now, I *never* want to go back to being that person again. That person was miserable. I couldn't feel joy and I didn't even know it."

I've written more on this subject in *Recovery from Parkinson's*.

If you determine that you are using self-induced pause, please read *Stuck on Pause* available online for free download at www.pdrecovery.com, or in hardcopy (book form) at JaniceHadlock.com.

This book has very detailed, specific instructions that will enable you to turn off this *psychological* behavior.

Can both pause or dissociation co-exist? A review

As mentioned at the beginning of this appendix, both pause and dissociation might be present at an injury site.

In this case, the person who's visualizing light or dark in his body, whichever is easier, *might* first see a motionless, heavy, or invisible situation when he gazes at a dark area: dissociation. However, after turning off the dissociation by mentally re-connecting with that area, he may discover that the area is *now* dark and agitated: pause. The underlying pause situation has been exposed, and can be addressed.

Or oppositely, his inner gaze *might* first reveal that some body part is dark and agitated. After turning off pause, the area is dark and heavy: dissociated, and able to respond to techniques that re-associate, reconnect.

Both self-induced dissociation and self-induced pause can be caused by the person *choosing* to avoid or *not* deal with the original trauma. They can both be thought of as mind-based, rather than biological, creations.

This means that there is *not* a one-size-fits-all "typical, biology-based" scenario to describe what the person might mentally have done while putting together his trauma-denial response.

If a person *chooses* to put his trauma on hold, all bets are off when trying to figure out whether pause or dissociation came first. He might have one, the other, or both.

Don't *worry* about whether dissociation or pause came first. Just treat whatever presents as dominant.

You can start your healing work by assuming that you are using basic dissociation and/or basic pause (as opposed to self-induced).

If the visualized area is dark and *immobile*, re-associate using the light and energy technique in this book.

If the visualized area is dark and is *agitated*, vibrating, or swirling, then use the techniques in the book *Stuck on Pause*.

Then, if the *other* pattern shows up. then treat the newly exposed pattern.

BUT THEN, if the dissociation and/or pause are treated and the body becomes full of light *but* five minutes later or the next day or week those body parts are dark again, then *self-induced* pause and/or *self-induced* dissociation is most likely the culprit.

The different types of trauma denial require different treatments. But whatever has been done can be undone.

As demonstrated in the golf cart case towards the beginning this appendix, a person can have an assortment of issues, including having both self-induced dissociation *and* pause, or any other combination. A person can even be *mildly* dissociated from his whole body and *extremely* dissociated from specific limbs. Anything is possible.

This next case study demonstrates this point. The point is that logical and neat labels of "one or the other" do not necessary exist when a person has decided to suppress his pain, his emotions and/or his past.

The final case study: self-induced pause *and* dissociation except while flying like an airplane

I had a patient who was using self-induced pause. He had severe, highly advanced Parkinson's disease. He could barely move. He could not feed himself or care for himself.

He perceived himself as being outside of his body. Inside his body, everything was dark. *But*, his neck and arms were darker and *more* dissociated than the rest of his body.

When, with eyes closed, he imagined he was looking at his body from the outside, most of it was approximately in the same place as his physical body. However, his *arms* were perceived as dead and withered, like blackened sticks, and sticking straight up in the air at a strange angle to his shoulders, unable to be lowered. His own mental image of his neck was that it was snapped, as if he'd died from a hanging. He had never noticed his weird arms and neck until I first asked him to imagine that he was looking around inside his body.

This person had both self-induced pause regarding his entire body *and* dissociation from his arms and neck. Most of his body was alive and on pause *but* his arms and neck had died.

From his out-of-body perspective, looking at himself, his actual physical body was a mere inanimate object with no significant amount of sensory function, an object that he could observe, unemotionally, from his paused vantage point of floating in space.

From this out-of-body perspective, he *could* temporarily imagine that most of his physical body was filled with light. However, when he did this, his imagined arms were still dark and withered. They still stuck upwards, out of his shoulders. And his neck was still broken.

And yet, for one time, and one time only, he was able to *temporarily* slide into a personality that *didn't* have pause by recalling how he'd felt inside when being a member of a famous dance troupe in his young adult years.

During this one-time event, he turned off his Parkinson's symptoms. He could move his whole body perfectly normally.

This not-unusual ability to slide out of pause when conditions are "exactly right" is described in detail in *Stuck on Pause.*

His one hour of normal movement occurred after I'd worked with him for about half an hour in his back yard. I was holding him up, encouraging him to pretend he was still a dancer (I held his shoulders and he shuffled in tiny steps while singing with me). While he alternated between singing and protesting he couldn't remember how to move, he suddenly began to trot in big circles, flapping his wings like a bird.

Gleeful at his sudden mobility, he held his arms out sideways and played at being an airplane, dipping and banking. He was radiant and laughing. Convinced that he had recovered from Parkinson's, he threw his arm over my shoulder and we danced the hora, kicking and swaying.

However, after about fifteen minutes of this, he turned to me and said, "I can't have actually recovered from Parkinson's so quickly, can I?" His body snapped back into utter rigidity. He had to be helped into the house, and his arms were once again pressed hard, rigid, against his torso. In his mind's eye, they were once again withered and black, sticking up in the air.

Curiously, he was pretty sure his feeling that he'd broken his neck had occurred when he was twenty, when he saw a *movie* in which a person was hanged by the neck.

He had no recall of any neck incident that had happened to him – but he remembered that the movie had profoundly affected him. At the time, he had been deeply disturbed, as if he'd awakened a memory of having been hung by the neck in a past lifetime.

The above example might seem over the top, but I can assure you, I've had patients, especially patients with Parkinson's, who've presented with even stranger ideas about where their "real" bodies actually are (miles away, in many cases) and what their various body parts are doing, and can nevertheless switch into absolute normalcy for a short time if doing something that they've decided is safe. And no two people have the same definition of "safe."

For example, I had one patient with highly advanced Parkinson's who could always move normally while doing the laundry, because "It's *always* a good thing to be making things clean." She would snap back into Parkinson's as soon as she turned away from the washing machine.

Case studies like this are *not* examples of a *rare* and freakish psychological type of Parkinson's, what some doctors refer to dismissively as "psychogenic parkinsonism."

Psychogenic parkinsonism is the diagnosis when a person, usually in response to a severe emotional shock, such as an elderly person's loss of a spouse, manifests tremoring, faint voice, rigidity, and other symptoms similar to those of shock – or those of Parkinson's. These cases usually clear up within a few days or a few months, which is why they are dismissed as "merely" psychogenic Parkinson's.

The truth is that *most* cases of Parkinson's have a psychogenic root.

Getting back to my point, unmedicated people with Parkinson's who can experience short-term spurts of normalcy in response to temporarily feeling truly safe are, in my experience, in the *vast majority* of the people with Parkinson's disease.

198

Idiopathic Parkinson's disease is, in most cases, a psychological syndrome. Whether it is held in place by dissociation, self-induced dissociation, pause, or self-induced pause, the sub-dermal electrical schematics that cause the symptoms of Parkinson's are an exact match for the sub-dermal electrical schematics of pause.

In the case of dissociation, the long-term electrical behaviors of an unhealed foot injury in just the right place (the second cuneiform bone) can snowball over decades and eventually lead to electrical behaviors that *mimic* those of pause.

In the case of pause, the electrical behaviors are to be expected, inasmuch as that's how the electrical currents do flow when a person is on pause or self-induced pause.

The problem, in Parkinson's, is that dissociation or pause hasn't been turned off. And in most cases, it hasn't been turned off for *psychological* reasons, not physical ones.

Getting back to the subject of cases where more than one type of problem is presenting and deciding which situation to treat first, treat whatever you think is the main thing presenting at the moment.

What you treat first doesn't really matter, in the big picture.

The nature of the more dominant problem (pause, dissociation, or even self-induced mindsets) can change in response to treatment: a different problem may come to the surface when the *first* dominant problem is cleared up.

Again, an area that is *dissociated* may turn out to be hiding an old injury that has triggered *pause*. And vice versa.

Don't worry about what, exactly, you might be doing mentally in terms of labeling.

A person on pause *or* dissociated *or* using self-induced behaviors might be dissociated from his whole body, some parts of his body, or even somewhat dissociated from the whole body but *extra*-dissociated from certain body parts or events related to those body parts. And he might have local areas on pause or be on body-wide pause. And don't worry about which location to deal with first. Deal with all of them, one at a time or in groups, whichever works best for you. You created the situation without formal instruction. You can un-create it in whatever way works best for you.

In general, if both pause and dissociation are presenting, as was demonstrated in the golf cart case, turn off pause before turning off dissociation. If, after turning these off, they return, they were most likely self-induced. Turn off the instructions that created the self-induced patterns.

First, do no harm

The main reason that these appendices have been included in this book on Yin Tui Na is because a person who is stuck on pause or who is using self-induced pause should not receive FSR treatment or any other kind of Yin Tui Na treatment until pause has been turned off.

Treating a person with FSR or other types of Yin Tui Na *if pause is present* can cause profound subconscious distress and confusion. It can lead to the formation or strengthening of a blocker personality. This is discussed in detail in the book *Stuck on Pause*.

That book has much more information on pause and diagnosing pause. This short appendix was included here to help point a person in the direction of *Stuck on Pause* if there is *any* indication that pause or self-induced pause is present.

If you are stuck on pause, then treating pause – permanently turning it off – is where you should start.

I have said elsewhere in this book that you should treat whatever the predominant problem is. In cases where a person is both dissociated and is stuck in pause mode, then pause must be treated first. If a person is *only* dissociated from injuries and is not stuck on pause, then choose whichever location seems to be causing the most trouble and start with that one.

For more instructions on determining if a person is stuck on pause, dissociated, or both, please read chapter 17 in the book *Recovery from Parkinson's*. This chapter discussing how to diagnose what type of PD (pause-based or dissociation-based) a person has. Most people have both pause-based and dissociation based. They will want to start their recovery work by turning off pause. They should only start working on the dissociation issue after pause has been turned off. Very often, when pause turns off, the dissociation goes away on its own: the old injury experiences the long suppressed pain and the healthy healing that has been put on hold due to the dissociation.

Treating dissociation, however, will NOT turn off pause mode, and can even make it more difficult to *ever* turn off pause.

So, if both are presenting, treat pause first.

drawings and photos

About the author

Dr. Janice Walton-Hadlock, DAOM (Doctor of Acupuncture and Oriental Medicine), LAc (Licensed Acupuncturist) has been a professor at Five Branches, an acupuncture college in Santa Cruz, California, since 1998.

She is the founder and director of research at the non-profit Parkinson's Recovery Project since 1997. See: www.pdrecovery.org.

Dr. Walton-Hadlock obtained her Doctoral degree in Acupuncture and Oriental Medicine at Five Branches in San Jose, CA, and her Master's degree in Chinese Medicine at Five Branches in Santa Cruz, CA. She earned a BA in Biology and also studied History of Science at University of California, Santa Cruz, in 1974.

Her research articles have been published in the peer-reviewed *American Journal of Acupuncture*, *The Journal of Chinese Medicine*, and other journals in the field. Her "commentary" on a piece of published research was published in the *New England Journal of Medicine*. She was the first non-MD acupuncturist to be accepted for publication in this journal.

She has lectured extensively, at home and abroad. Continuing education credits from her videotaped lectures are available at the Eastern Currents Continuing Education program, EasternCurrents.ca.

She brings to her study of Chinese medicine a lifetime passion for ancient languages, modern physics, and world scriptures ancient and modern.

Other books by Janice Hadlock

Hacking Chinese Medicine
Tracking the Dragon: Advanced Channel Theory
Stuck on Pause*
Recovery from Parkinson's *
Medications of Parkinson's Disease or Once Upon a Pill: patient experiences
   with dopamine-enhancing drugs and supplements. #

————

Books are available at JaniceHadlock.com.

In Canada, ordering through EasternCurrents.ca will get you a better price on shipping. That address says .ca, *not* .com. The .ca = Canada

* also available for *free* download at www.pdrecovery.org, the website for the non-profit Parkinson's Recovery Project

not available in hard-copy because, at over 700 8" x 11" pages, it is too massive for paperback edition. *Only* available for *free* download at www.pdrecovery.org.